AF764444

SURGERY - PROCEDURES, COMPLICATIONS, AND RESULTS

PROSTATECTOMIES

PROCEDURES, BENEFITS AND POTENTIAL COMPLICATIONS

SURGERY - PROCEDURES, COMPLICATIONS, AND RESULTS

Additional books in this series can be found on Nova's website under the Series tab.

Additional e-books in this series can be found on Nova's website under the e-book tab.

PUBLIC HEALTH IN THE 21ST CENTURY

Additional books in this series can be found on Nova's website under the Series tab.

Additional e-books in this series can be found on Nova's website under the e-book tab.

SURGERY - PROCEDURES, COMPLICATIONS, AND RESULTS

PROSTATECTOMIES

PROCEDURES, BENEFITS AND POTENTIAL COMPLICATIONS

HENRIQUE MAYA ALVELOS
AND
YARA GRÃO IZIDORO
EDITORS

Nova Science Publishers, Inc.
New York

Copyright © 2012 by Nova Science Publishers, Inc.

All rights reserved. No part of this book may be reproduced, stored in a retrieval system or transmitted in any form or by any means: electronic, electrostatic, magnetic, tape, mechanical photocopying, recording or otherwise without the written permission of the Publisher.

For permission to use material from this book please contact us:
Telephone 631-231-7269; Fax 631-231-8175
Web Site: http://www.novapublishers.com

NOTICE TO THE READER

The Publisher has taken reasonable care in the preparation of this book, but makes no expressed or implied warranty of any kind and assumes no responsibility for any errors or omissions. No liability is assumed for incidental or consequential damages in connection with or arising out of information contained in this book. The Publisher shall not be liable for any special, consequential, or exemplary damages resulting, in whole or in part, from the readers' use of, or reliance upon, this material. Any parts of this book based on government reports are so indicated and copyright is claimed for those parts to the extent applicable to compilations of such works.

Independent verification should be sought for any data, advice or recommendations contained in this book. In addition, no responsibility is assumed by the publisher for any injury and/or damage to persons or property arising from any methods, products, instructions, ideas or otherwise contained in this publication.

This publication is designed to provide accurate and authoritative information with regard to the subject matter covered herein. It is sold with the clear understanding that the Publisher is not engaged in rendering legal or any other professional services. If legal or any other expert assistance is required, the services of a competent person should be sought. FROM A DECLARATION OF PARTICIPANTS JOINTLY ADOPTED BY A COMMITTEE OF THE AMERICAN BAR ASSOCIATION AND A COMMITTEE OF PUBLISHERS.

Additional color graphics may be available in the e-book version of this book.

Library of Congress Cataloging-in-Publication Data

ISBN: 978-1-62081-077-4

Published by Nova Science Publishers, Inc. † New York

Contents

Preface

In this book, the authors present current research in the study of the procedures, benefits and potential complications of prostatectomies. Topics discussed include suprapubic prostatecomy for benign prostatic hyperplasia; management of post-prostatectomy incontinence; biochemical recurrence following radical prostatectomy; techniques for neuro-vascular bundle preservation; and extraperitoneal endoscopic radical prostatectomy techniques.

Chapter I - Among other therapies for the localized prostate cancer, radical prostatectomy continues to play a prominent role and to be the gold standard in comparison with novel emerging treatments. The rationale of removing the malignant tumor together with the involved organ is as ancient as medicine itself. There is still no uniformly accepted consensus on indications and contraindications for radical removal of the prostate (radical prostatectomy). As well, there is still ongoing discussion as to the best approach to perform the operation. The argument is mainly held between advocates of time honored anatomic radical retropubic prostatectomy and supporters of robot-assisted laparoscopic radical prostatectomy. In this chapter the authors will extensively elaborate on the benefits and drawbacks of these two methods, as well as other, less popular approaches (laparoscopic radical prostatectomy, perineal radical prostatectomy). The authors will discuss these techniques in detail. Will also touch on the subject of prostatectomy for benign prostate hyperplasia.

Chapter II - Suprapubic prostatectomy for benign prostatic hyperplasia (BPH) remains a viable option in the surgical treatment of BPH for the adequately selected patients and is the predominant method of surgical treatment of BPH in the developing world. One of the discouraging aspects of suprapubic prostatectomy is the frequent and significant hemorrhage that can be encountered. Controlling hemorrhage after suprapubic prostatectomy has always been a point of research from the time this method of surgery was developed. At present time it can be said that controlling hemostasis is one of the key factors to a safe and successful outcome of suprapubic prostatectomy. The difficulties encountered over the years in achieving good hemostasis has continued to frustrate many urologists involved in doing this surgery. In this paper the authors give a brief history of methods previously used to achieve hemostasis during suprapubic prostatectomy and then highlight our method of hemostasis which in our experience has been very effective in controlling bleeding during suprapubic prostatectomy.

Chapter III - Urinary incontinence can occur after surgery for benign and malignant diseases of the prostate, including radical prostatectomy and endoscopic prostate surgery. Most often the incontinence is mild or transient, however if it is severe or persists, the incontinence can have detrimental effects on patient's quality of life. Thorough evaluation of the patient with a detailed history, physical examination, and diagnostic studies is necessary to formulate the diagnosis and tailor the treatment. The focus of this chapter is on the evaluation and treatment of post-prostatectomy stress urinary incontinence.

Chapter IV - *Introduction*: The surgical treatment of prostate cancer has evolved rapidly, driven by technological advances that have made minimally-invasive prostatectomy feasible. The contemporary surgical approaches are laparoscopic radical prostatectomy and robot-assisted laparoscopic radical prostatectomy that are considered standard modalities across North America, Europe and other reference centers. Despite the widespread adoption of these new techniques there are few robust studies directly comparing the results of these techniques with the standard open radical prostatectomy. This review aim to discuss the current status of minimally- invasive prostatectomy focusing on peri-operative, oncological and functional outcomes, costs and availability in different centers worldwide. *Matherial and methods*: Analysis of published literature in PUBMED and google academic utilizing laparoscopic radical prostatectomy and robotic radical prostatectomy as key words. Peri-operative data ,oncological control, continence and potency rates, costs and availability in several centers around the world were compared.

Chapter V - The risk of cancer recurrence after radical prostatectomy can be estimated using nomograms based on validated prognostic factors. Follow-up can then be tailored to a patient's risk. The diagnosis of recurrence after radical prostatectomy is made when the PSA is greater than 0.2ng/ml. After recurrence, the great dilemma is to determine whether the recurrence is localized or systemic. This can be determined by a variety of imaging modalities and examination of prostatectomy characteristics and PSA kinetics. Management of a recurrence can be expectant or therapy with salvage radiotherapy or androgen ablation therapy depending on the likelihood of localized disease, patient health and expectations.

Chapter VI - Radical prostatectomy (RP) is the gold standard treatment for localized prostate cancer. Since excellent survival rates are reported with this therapeutic approach, functionality is the next major concern nowadays. Sexual potency is a mayor issue, so neuro-vascular bundle (NVB) preservation is the rule when indicated. Walsh published the first anatomical nerve-sparing technique for radical prostatectomy. He described detailed anatomy of the cavernous nerves and their distribution around the prostate. He also showed how to avoid neural injury by incising the lateral pelvic fascia anterior to the NVB and dividing the lateral pedicles closely to the prostate. Further improvements in the detail of the periprostatic neural anatomy have been accomplished. Anterior and posterior branches of the NVB have been defined, as well as the predominant NVB and accessory neural pathways. Finally, although the vast majority of nerves are found in the rectolateral sides of the prostate, a significant amount of nerve bundles are found in superior lateral portions. Meticulous anatomy descriptions and technological advances such as surgical magnification (loupes), laparoscopy and robot assisted surgery have improved NVB preservation and different techniques have been described.

Chapter VII - Laparoscopic and robotic assisted radical prostatectomies are continuous developing techniques, with feasibility and reproducibility demonstrated worldwide. Low morbidity and excellent functional and oncological outcomes can be achieved, although learning curve without robotic assistance is longer. The majority of centers that employ this technique have preferred transperitoneal access. Few groups prefer endoscopic extra peritoneal route but this surgical access is currently receiving a higher acceptance. The authors herein review the improvements in their personal technique reporting current experience with endoscopic extra peritoneal radical prostatectomy (EEERP) as a first line therapy for localized prostate cancer.

Chapter VIII - Radical prostatectomy is the most widely applied treatment for localized prostate cancer. Postoperative PSA levels are expected to be close to zero and PSA levels above 0.2 ng/dL generally characterize recurrence. However, there is no consensual definition for PSA levels to define cure after radical prostatectomy yet. The aim of the present study was to evaluate post prostatectomy PSA level and its association with prostate cancer relapse. *Methods:* A hundred and six men (median=64.0±6.9 years, range 49-80 years) with localized prostate cancer underwent radical retropubic prostatectomy were followed between 1996 and 2006, for a minimum 24-month follow up (mean 46.5 months). Postoperative ultrasensitive PSA levels were assessed after 30 days, every 3 months for the first two years and twice a year thereafter. Patients were divided in four groups according to postoperative PSA nadir: Group 1 (<0.04 ng/dL); group 2 (0.04-0.09 ng/dL); group 3 (0.09 –0.2 ng/dL); and group 4 (>0.2 ng/dL).

In: Prostatectomies
Editors: H. Alvelos and Y. Izidoro
ISBN: 978-1- 62081-077-4
© 2012 Nova Science Publishers, Inc.

Chapter I

Prostatectomies: Procedures, Benefits and Potential Complications

Vladimir Yutkin, Ana Maria Autran and Jonathan Izawa
University of Western Ontario, Uro-Oncology Fellowship Program, London, Canada

Abstract

Among other therapies for the localized prostate cancer, radical prostatectomy continues to play a prominent role and to be the gold standard in comparison with novel emerging treatments. The rationale of removing the malignant tumor together with the involved organ is as ancient as medicine itself. There is still no uniformly accepted consensus on indications and contraindications for radical removal of the prostate (radical prostatectomy). As well, there is still ongoing discussion as to the best approach to perform the operation. The argument is mainly held between advocates of time honored anatomic radical retropubic prostatectomy and supporters of robot-assisted laparoscopic radical prostatectomy. In this chapter we will extensively elaborate on the benefits and drawbacks of these two methods, as well as other, less popular approaches (laparoscopic radical prostatectomy, perineal radical prostatectomy). We will discuss these techniques in detail. We will also touch on the subject of prostatectomy for benign prostate hyperplasia.

Furthermore, we will comment on the outcomes, long and short-term complications and side effects of every approach and compare them with each other, as well as with alternative techniques of minimally invasive surgery including cryoablation of prostate and high intensity focused ultrasound. In addition, we will concentrate on follow-up of prostate cancer after radical prostatectomy, definitions of failure, and different indications for adjuvant and salvage treatment after the operation given the diverse stages of the disease. Finally, we will mention various approaches to cope with complications and side effects of prostatectomy and their influence on quality of life issues.

Introduction

The prostate is a small accessory gland in the male genito-urinary system, which receives disproportionally high attention, relatively to its size. The main function of the gland in a healthy male is to produce the part of seminal fluid that is rich in enzymes, especially proteases that assist in semen liquefaction in female genital tract thus promoting adequate sperm movement toward the oocyte. During the first 3 decades of life diseases of the prostate are rare, but become increasingly frequent with aging. In the United States benign prostatic hyperplasia (BPH) is among the 10 most prevalent diseases in men older than 50 years of age in terms of the morbidity and associated costs [1]. In the majority of cases, BPH is managed conservatively with only minority of the patients requiring surgery that is usually due to worsening voiding symptoms or the inability to urinate. Other benign conditions that may involve the prostate are usually inflammatory or of an infectious origin.

Prostate Adenocarcinoma and Its Surgical Treatment

Prostate adenocarcinoma is the most common non-skin cancer in men both in US [2] and in Europe [3]. As a salient feature of many malignancies, at the beginning the disease has an insidious course, causing no appreciable symptoms. Also, similar to other malignancies, this is the best window of opportunity with the highest chance for cure. That is why the diagnosis of curable prostate cancer relies on screening and early diagnosis. This is a controversial topic, the discussion of which is beyond the scope of this chapter.

According to 2010 NCCN Guidelines [4], the following options are available to patient and physician when localized prostate cancer is diagnosed: active surveillance, radiation therapy (both external beam and brachytherapy) and radical prostatectomy. The optimal management choice depends on the disease features and patient characteristics.

One of the first descriptions of the radical removal of the prostate was described by Dr. H.H. Young in 1905 [5]. In that era it was a very difficult operation with high mortality and morbidity invariably leaving the patients with severe urinary incontinence and total erectile dysfunction. Nevertheless, with numerous modifications that were introduced over the century, the open radical prostatectomy remains the gold standard in the management of the localized prostate cancer. The most credit in shaping the contemporary approach to radical retropubic prostatectomy (RRP) belongs to Dr. Patrick C. Walsh, especially for understanding the precise anatomy of the pelvis and the preservation of erectile function [6]. Both laparoscopic and robot assisted approaches were shaped according to the open approach [6].

Preoperative Work-Up

Despite the emergence of trans-rectal ultrasound (TRUS) and magnetic resonance imaging (MRI), the digital rectal examination (DRE) remains an invaluable tool for assessment of tumor extent and possible involvement of adjacent tissues.

There is usually no need in extensive preoperative imaging, unless there is a significant likelihood of metastatic disease, which is usually indicated by PSA level over 20 ng/ml and/or Gleason score over 7. In these cases computed tomography and bone scintigraphy are performed. MRI imaging of the prostate using the endorectal coil [7] may be to be superior in the diagnosis of the extra-prostatic extension of the cancer.

The widely accepted contraindications for surgery include life expectancy of less than 15 years and/or the presence of metastatic disease.

Usually, the surgery is delayed for at least 6 weeks after TRUS-guided needle prostate biopsy in order to allow the inflammatory processes and hematomas to resolve, restoring the normal tissue plains.

Adequate measures to prevent intraoperative or postoperative deep vein thromboembolism should be undertaken (i.e. pneumatic compression stockings and low-molecular weight heparin). According to the American Urological Association (AUA) best practice guidelines, preoperative antibiotic treatment is limited to 24 hours with first or second generation cephalosporin or an aminoglycoside in combination with metronidazole or clindamycin [8].

The operation is performed under general or regional anesthesia.

Special Instruments

The only special instruments that are needed in this procedure are the self-retaining Balfour or Omni retractor with malleable and grooved blades, fiber optic head-light and magnification loupes with at least x2.5 power.

Procedure

The patient is placed supine, prepped and draped in the usual way. Some surgeons prefer the dorsal lithotomy position. An 18-20F Foley catheter is inserted into the bladder and the balloon is inflated to 20-30 ml. The 10 cm midline incision is made well below the umbilicus to the pubic bone through the skin and fascia, and muscles are separated at the midline without entering the peritoneum. The retropubic space of Retzius is entered and dissected laterally to the level of bifurcation of the common iliac vessels. The self-retaining retractor is placed with malleable blade retracting the bladder and peritoneal content superiorly. At this stage the pelvic lymph node dissection is done. The limits of the dissection are bifurcation of common iliac vessels superiorly, urinary bladder medially, to the pelvic side wall laterally (usually sparing the lymphatics overlying the external iliac artery) and to the internal opening of the femoral canal inferiorly. Great care is taken not to injure the obturator nerve during this dissection. The procedure is performed using right angle clamp, Metzenbaum scissors, Debakey or Russian forceps and clips. The fat tissue overlying the anterior surface of the prostate is also removed exposing the superficial dorsal vein and puboprostatic ligaments, and may be sent as separate sample, as it may contain lymph nodes in up to 15% of patients [9]. Next, the endopelvic fascia is opened bilaterally just lateral to the arcus tendineus of levator ani muscle. After the incision, the muscle fibers of the levator ani are swept laterally thus exposing the angle between prostate and rectum and the location of neuro-vascular bundle (NVB). Then, the pubo-prostatic ligaments are divided carefully with Metzenbaum scissors to the point where the apex of the prostate is exposed. The deep dorsal vein complex (DVC) is oversewn with one or two figure-of-eight 2-0 absorbable sutures. This suture is placed just distal to the prostate apex. Another figure of eight suture is placed proximal to bladder neck to prevent the back bleeding which can be quite substantial. After that, the DVC can be safely divided immediately distal to the apex of the prostate to the level of urethra. When the urethra is exposed, the right angle clamp is insinuated beneath it and the upper half of the urethra is divided while the urethral catheter is exposed. Next, the balloon of the catheter is emptied and the catheter is pulled back till the posterior wall of the urethra is exposed. The 6 anastomotic sutures are placed with 2-0 monocryl suture and the urethra is divided completely. After this, the posterior wall of striated sphincter complex is divided, taking care not to damage the NVB which is sometimes connected to the prostate apex by small apical vessel. The NVB is located between the two layers of lateral pelvic fascia: the levator ani fascia laterally, which forms the arcus tendineus and prostatic fascia medially. In order to preserve the NVB the dissection is best performed inter-fascially (i.e. between these two fascial layers). The superficial layer, levator fascia, is opened bluntly with fine right angle clamp along the antero-lateral surface of the prostate. The small vessels between NVB and prostate are ligated or clipped and the bundles are dissected from the prostate up to the level of lateral pedicle. Care is taken not to use the electro-cautery during the dissection of NVB, as it has been shown to have both short and long term detrimental effects on the cavernous nerve tissue [10].

After two thirds of the prostate length is dissected retrogradely, Denonvillier's fascia is opened at the midline and the ampullae of vasa deferentia are dissected out and divided following by dissection of seminal vesicles. It should be remembered that on the postero-lateral surface of the seminal vesicle the pelvic nervous plexus is located. The small arterial branches are located at the tips of seminal vesicles and should be controlled prospectively. As the seminal vesicles are freed from the surrounding tissues, the lateral pedicle is ligated and divided, leaving the prostate connected to the bladder only by the bladder neck. This is opened at the anterior prostato-vesical junction. The rest of the bladder neck is divided and prostate is removed after identifying the ureteral orifices. After the prostate is removed, the prostate bed is inspected for the possible bleeding sources, which are meticulously controlled with clips or ligated. No cautery is used in the proximity of the NVB or pelvic autonomic plexus. The removal of the prostate usually leaves the bladder neck with an opening that is much larger than the diameter of the membranous urethra, so before performing the anastomosis, tailoring of the bladder neck is accomplished with absorbable suture, usually in the "tennis racquet" fashion. If ureteral catheters were placed upon opening the bladder neck, they are removed at this point. It is convenient to evert the bladder mucosa with fine absorbable interrupted sutures to potentially minimize vesico-urethral anastomotic contracture formation.

The vesico-urethral anastomosis is most often performed with 6 2-0 monocryl sutures, using a urethral catheter or retractable urethral sound to help identify the urethral mucosa, although the continuous anastomosis has been described, allowing the catheter removal as soon as 48 hours post-operatively [11]. The anastomosis should be water tight and tension free. If there is any doubt in its quality, it is better to take the whole anastomosis down and re-do it, because the possible complications of a faulty anastomosis may be lifelong incontinence or anastomotic strictures. After it is completed, the balloon of the urethral catheter is inflated and most surgeons place a closed suction drain through separate stab wound to the vicinity of the anastomosis. If a surgeon has extensive experience and excellent results showing a negligible risk of anastomotic leak or lymphocele formation, it is reasonable to forgo a drain.

Postoperative Care

The preoperative medications are resumed after a patient is discharged from the acute postoperative care unit; the pain management usually consists of ketorolac and is aimed at early ambulation. The patient usually can be discharged from the hospital on the second postoperative day with usual restrictions on weight lifting. If placed, the pelvic drain is removed on post-operative day 1 or 2, depending on the amount of the drainage. The urethral catheter is left indwelling for five to 14 days, depending on the anastomosis technique and surgeon preference. If the removal of the catheter is planned at postoperative day 10 or later, no cystogram is required prior to removal to ensure integrity of the vesico-urethral anastomosis.

Complications

Intraoperative Complications

- *Bleeding:* Intraoperative bleeding occurs usually from the DVC, which should be controlled prior to its division; otherwise the precise apical dissection and NVB preservation might be very difficult, aside the fact that the patient may lose blood unnecessarily. Other potential sources of bleeding may be iliac vessels that can be injured inadvertently during the lymph node dissection.

- *Rectal injury:* This is relatively rare complication, occurring in less than 1% of patients [12], but may be more common in previously irradiated patients. The most important thing in managing it is in its timely recognition. If the injury is recognized during the operation, it should be closed primarily in two layers with excellent results [12], while delayed recognition due to recto-vesical or recto-urethral fistula always necessitates diverting ileostomy and delayed repair of the fistula.
- *Ureteral injury:* This rare complication is can be prevented by selective intraoperative stenting of both ureters, as previously described. If it happens, the uretero-neocystostomy over the ureteral stent should be performed after prostate removal and before urethra-bladder anastomosis.
- *Obturator nerve injury:* It is very rare event, that may occur during the dissection of the obturator lymph nodes, and if the trans-section is recognized, it should be repaired by reapproximation with fine non-absorbable sutures immediately [13], expecting good functional results.

Early Post-Operative Complications

Infection is a rare postoperative complication if the routine periprocedural measures to prevent it are performed. Persistent drainage of urine from the suction drain may occur if the vesico-urethral anastomosis or bladder neck reconstruction is leaking, but these are also relatively rate complications.

The best policy in this case is to provide maximal drainage of the urine from the bladder in order to minimize the leakage and to prevent an establishment of the fistula tract. After the leak stops, it is prudent to perform a cystogram prior to catheter removal.

The lymphatic drainage can be quite substantial after pelvic lymph node dissection, but it almost always eventually stops. Sometimes canceling the vacuum from the drainage system may hasten the recovery.Delayed bleeding from the prostate bed or DVC may cause hypotension and require blood transfusions.

The risk should be less than 5%. If it happens, repeat exploration, evacuating the pelvic hematoma should be considered, as conservative management may result in post-operative vesico-urethral anastomotic strictures [14].

Late Post-Operative Complications

- *Erectile dysfunction:* The prevalence of the erectile dysfunction after prostatectomy may reach 60-65% even if the nerve sparing approach is implemented [15], [16]. The early rehabilitation of the erectile function postoperatively may be beneficial, as shown in animal studies and some human trials using phosphodiesterase-5 inhibitors early after surgery [17].
- *Urinary incontinence*: Up to 20% of patients after radical prostatectomy may be dissatisfied with their urinary continence [16], although in one surgeon series the results can be as good as 93% satisfaction [18]. The severity may range from losing a few drops of urine a day to total incontinence. The improvement usually takes place during the 6-12 months following the operation and therefore patients should wait beyond this period before undertaking surgical procedures in an attempt to alleviate their incontinence.
- *Anastomotic (bladder neck) contracture*: This particular stricture, occurs in 0-10% of patients [19]. This usually develops after one to two months following the procedure. Patients will report gradual improvement in urinary incontinence but worsening of the urinary stream. The factors that predispose for development of this complication are poor approximation or mucosal surfaces during the vesico-urethral anastomosis, postoperative urinary extravasation and pelvic/ peri-anastamotic hematoma that was not drained [14].

Follow Up after Radical Prostatectomy

Serum PSA is very precise tumor marker after radical prostatectomy, as no residual prostate tissue or prostate cancer should be present. The usual follow up consists of serial PSA measurements, where a PSA level above 0.2 ng/ml invariably indicates prostate cancer recurrence (biochemical recurrence) [20].

The timing of PSA recurrence and rate of its rise help determine a local versus metastatic recurrence, but the discussion on this topic is beyond the scope of this chapter.

Radical Perineal Prostatectomy

The radical perineal prostatectomy (RPP) is the oldest means of prostate resection and at one time was the standard of care for surgical treatment of localized prostate cancer [5, 21]. However, the procedure became less popular during 1970´s after Walsh and Donker demonstrated the advantages of a nerve-sparing technique using a retropubic approach [22].

Indications and Contraindications

The indications for use of RPP are identical to radical retropubic prostatectomy. The perineal route may be beneficial in men after previous retropubic surgery with obscured surgical planes (i.e. bilateral hernioplasty with synthetic mesh, renal transplantation, pelvic vascular surgery) or in extremely obese patients. RPP is considered in patients not requiring a pelvic lymph node dissection, as performing this procedure by perineal approach is virtually impossible. Alternatively, in patients with high risk of lymph node involvement, the dissection can be performed as a separate procedure via a laparoscopic approach [23]. The RPP is less advocated in men with previous prostate surgery and history of ankylosis of the hip due to use of an exaggerated lithotomy position during the procedure. The procedure can also be difficult in patients with prostate larger than 100 grams and a narrow pelvis [24, 25].

Special Instruments [21]

The instruments required include curved and straight Lowsley retractors, notched Young bulb retractor, Duval clamp and self-retaining retractor (e.g. Bookwalter).

Procedure

The patient is placed in exaggerated lithotomy position in order to get proper access to perineum. Next, the curved Lowsley retractor is inserted through the urethra into the bladder and its blades are opened. This maneuver facilitates moving the prostate in the operative field. Inverted U incision is made through the skin and the subcutaneous tissues of the perineum, dividing the central tendon of the perineum, aiming to the plane between the external anal sphincter and the bulbo-cavernosus muscle. When the prostate apex is reached, it is dissected from the levator any muscle fibers laterally and sharply from the recto-urethralis muscle dorsally.

Great care should be taken at this stage, as the rectum is usually tented up ventrally and can be easily injured. After the levator ani and the rectum are dissected off the prostate, the entire dorsal prostatic surface can be seen. Now the posterior layer of Denonvilliers' fascia is incised and dissected off the prostate laterally together with NVB if nerve-sparing approach is attempted. Similarly to retropubic approach, excessive traction and electro-cautery are avoided in vicinity of NVB.

Next, the Denonvilliers' fascia is stripped from the vasa deferentia and seminal vesicles which are then dissected free of surrounding tissues using hemoclips or ligatures for hemostatis due to proximity of autonomic nervous plexus. Then the prostatic pedicles are controlled and the bladder neck is dissected circumferentially without dividing it. Next, the membranous urethra is divided dorsally and the curved Lowsley retractor is replaced with the straight one and the distal urethra is catheterized with a catheter to help with the upward traction.

Now the ventral wall of the urethra is divided, DVC is pushed up bluntly and pubo-prostatic ligaments are sectioned. The prostate is dissected on its ventral surface towards the bladder neck, which is then divided. Like in retropubic approach, the ureteral orifices should be identified prior to dividing the posterior bladder neck. The prostate is removed and bladder neck reconstruction with vesico-urethral anastomosis are performed over urethral catheter, similar to retropubic approach. Postoperative care is virtually the same as in retropubic approach.

Comparison of RRP and RPP

The only unique complication of RPP is neuropraxia of sural nerve and compartment syndrome due to exaggerated lithotomy position. Price et al [26] reported that 43 of 111 patients experienced some degree of lower extremity neuropraxia. The incidence of rectal injury during the RPP was also reported to be higher than in RRP [27]. In terms of oncological and functional outcomes both open approaches have similar results. Salomon et al [28] reported PSMs rates of 17% in RPP group vs. 12% in RRP patients. Similarly, May et al [29] reported comparable overall positive surgical margins rates with apical positive margins significantly less common in the RPP group (5.8 vs. 17.2% in RPP vs. RRP, respectively). Recently Prasad et al [30] found that RPP compares favorably vs. RRP in terms of requirement of the adjuvant treatment: 4.9% vs. 6.9%, respectively. Relative to the retropubic approach the blood loss in RPP has been reported as being less extensive [28, 31], but is highly surgeon and series specific, as shown by the transfusion rates reported: between 0.3 to 33% [27, 30].

Minimally Invasive Surgical Techniques in the Treatment of the Prostate Cancer

In the quest for further improvement of radical prostatectomy oncological and especially functional outcomes, minimally invasive approaches to the procedure were developed, i.e. purely laparoscopic (LRP) and robotic assisted laparoscopic prostatectomy (RALP). The first report of LRP was made in 1992 by Schuessler et al [32], the technique being further modified in European centers [33, 34].

The minimally invasive technique was aimed on reducing blood loss and on shortening the patients' recovery. However, LRP demonstrated to be a complex procedure requiring a highly skilled laparoscopic surgeon and had a long learning curve.

The robotic assisted technique came shortly thereafter [35, 36] and brought a 3-dimentional view, x10 magnification and a unique mimicking of human hand and wrist on the working end of the instrument. These attributes allowed a shorter learning curve, much better ergonomics for the surgeon and gained immediate popularity despite the lack of data proving it provides better outcomes for patients.

Technically, the laparoscopic procedures by either method is very similar, thus we will describe them together. It should be mentioned, that the RRP had major influence on shaping and developing the laparoscopic procedures.

Indications and Preoperative Work-Up

These are virtually the same as in the open approach.

Special Instruments

In the case of RALP, there is a need in a specialized robotic system (i.e. *da Vinci®* surgical system (Intuitive Surgical, Sunnyvale, CA), which consists of a surgeon´s console and a patient-side cart with three or four interactive robotic arms If the LRP is contemplated, then the standard set of laparoscopy instruments is needed.

Procedure

The patient is placed supine in steep Trandelenburg position and after induction of anesthesia the legs are spread to allow the docking of the robot's patient cart and the access to perineum.

The pneumoperitoneum is achieved and working ports are introduced. In the case of robotic approach with 4-arm machine, 6 ports are usually placed: four for robot arms and 2 for assistant. If the LRP is performed, 5 ports are usually enough. The most prevalent approach for both procedures is transperitoneal antegrade resection. The first step is dissecting the bladder off the anterior abdominal wall and gaining the access to the retropubic space of Retzius. Next, the endopelvic fascia is opened, very much like in RRP, following by division of pubo-prostatic ligaments and ligation of the dorsal vein complex. The next step is division of the bladder neck at the prostate-bladder junction first anteriorly and then posteriorly, entering the plane between the prostate capsule and the bladder. Immediately after that the vasa deferentia are encountered, dissected free from surrounding tissue and divided, following by dissecting the seminal vesicles from their tip toward the base. After this the NVBs dissected off the gland and prostate pedicles dissected and divided. Again, similar to the open approach, the dissection around the seminal vesicles and NVBs is performed a-thermally. After these steps the prostate is left attached only by the DVC and urethra, which are sequentially divided and the specimen is left inside the special bag until the end of the procedure. The tailoring of the bladder neck is performed if needed and vesico-urethral anastomosis is performed using continuous monocryl suture. This continuous suturing technique allows removing urethral catheter after 3-5 days.

Postoperative Management

The minimally invasive approach has been shown to reduce the postoperative pain, and may allow an earlier hospital discharge [37], although with considerably higher direct costs. At our center, we have observed that hospital discharge is equivalent between RRP and RALP.

Complications

- *Bleeding:*Due to the reduced pressure gradient between the blood vasculature and the peritoneal cavity after achieving pneumo-peritoneum, the blood loss may be considerably lower with minimally advanced techniques [38], compared to the open prostatectomy. Again, this is highly dependent upon the surgeon performing the radical prostatectomy and the patient characteristics.
- *Erectile dysfunction:* Several studies have established that recovery of the erectile function after radical prostatectomy depends on multiple factors, including the status before the operation, the operative technique and the postoperative management [39]. Reportedly, the minimally invasive approach may lessen the damage to the NVB because the dissection occurs in an antegrade fashion reducing traction on the nerves; better vision allows more precise dissection preventing inadvertent incision or incorporation into suture or clip [40]. A progressive improvement in terms of erectile function recovery rates has been observed along the follow-up in multiple series. Thus, at 12 months between 20 and 97% of patients report sexual intercourse after nerve sparing technique [40]. Thus far, there is no definitive data showing one technique offers consistently better erectile function rates. Surgeon and patient characteristics remain critical factors.
- *Incontinence:*It is difficult to determine whether minimally invasive approach is superior in terms of recovery of urinary continence based on the current literature, but the long term the results are very similar [38, 41].

Oncological Outcomes

Several studies have suggested that a minimally invasive approach offers at least similar oncologic outcomes compared to open procedure, although to our knowledge, no randomized controlled trials of these procedures have been completed. Currently, limited long term oncologic control dates are available for LRP and RALP, thus most of the studies focus on assessing the PSM. Margin status is an important independent predictor of disease recurrence after radical prostatectomy and therefore a measure of treatment efficacy. In robotic surgery, the surgeon has the theoretical advantage of an enhanced ability to identify surgical dissection planes, hopefully leading to lower PSM. However, the lack of intra-operative tactile sensation during the procedure is sometimes cited as a drawback, inherent with robotics. In a multicenter study on 8095 patients who underwent RALP [42] the overall PSM rate was 15.7%. The PSM rate revealed after RRP and LRP found in critical review of literature: 24 and 21.3%, respectively [43]. Due to patient and surgeon differences, and the lack of a randomized trial, one cannot directly compare these results.

Minimallylly Invasive Local Ablative Techniques in the Treatment of Localized Prostate Cancer

Minimally invasive local therapies such as cryotherapy of the prostate and more recently high intensity focused ultrasound (HIFU) have emerged as alternatives in gland ablative therapies for localized prostate cancer, showing encouraging results in terms of morbidity rates and cancer control in the short term.

Cryotherapy

The technique was introduced in the 1960´s [44], and was used initially with open approach in the treatment of benign and malignant prostate conditions; it was approved as a primary therapy for the prostate cancer by the FDA in 1999.

Treatment Principles

Different mechanisms of cell death have been implicated in cryotherapy. A key mechanism is the induction of ice crystals within the prostate cancer cells which results in physical disruption of the cells. Crystallization and cellular death begin when the temperature falls below 0°C within the cells. However, adequate tissue destruction and resultant coagulative necrosis requires significantly lower temperatures of at least -40°C.

Ideally, once temperatures reach – 40°C, the cells would break down to allow maximal destruction of the cellular matrix, resulting in cellular death. Intracellular changes such as protein denaturation damages, electrolyte and osmotic changes are also part of the cytocidal process. At the extracellular level, thrombosis of the microvasculature and tissue matrix destruction also contribute to a damage to the prostate gland. The cooling gas is delivered to the gland through the specially designed probes. These probes utilize the Joule-Thompson principle where gases which were previously compressed are allowed to expand, resulting in an associated temperature change. Some gases decrease their temperature with expansion (e.g. Argon, resulting in freezing) while others increase their temperature (e.g. Helium, resulting in warming). [45].

Preoperative Work-Up, Indications

These are virtually the same as radical prostatectomy. In addition, cryotherapy has been used as a salvage procedure due to cancer recurrent after radiation therapy [46].

Special Instruments and Equipment

A TRUS cryogenic system is equipped with template, stands, warming probes, urethral warming device and thermocouples.

Procedure

After induction of anesthesia the patient is placed in lithotomy position; urethral catheter is inserted into the bladder and clamped to facilitate the prostate gland visualization on TRUS. The brachytherapy-like template on adaptive cradle is mounted on the table and the TRUS probe secured to it and inserted into the rectum. The prostate is visualized and measured and the treatment is planned. The cooling probes together with thermocouples are inserted through the perineum into the gland under the TRUS guidance. Prior to initiating the treatment the urethral catheter is exchanged to the urethral warming device. Usually two freeze-thaw cycles are performed [47] with rapid freezing and slow thawing under continuous monitoring of the tissue temperature with the thermocouples.

Postoperative Management

The patient usually can be discharged from the hospital on the same or the next day after the surgery. The urethral catheter is removed after 2-5 days.

Complications

- *Urinary retention.* Can be caused by the swelling of the gland secondary to the treatment. It is usually temporary phenomenon and is treated by indwelling urethral catheter.
- *Fistula formation.* During early stages of the development of the cryosurgery technique, this was relatively common complication. This is not the case with introduction of the new technologies, including vigorous temperature monitoring and high resolution TRUS. The recent reported incidence is not higher than in the radical prostatectomy [48]: between 0 to 0.5%.
- *Erectile dysfunction.* Due to the inclusion of both NVB into the ice ball, impotence is a very common sequela of this treatment, reaching 95% of the patients [49].
- *Incontinence.* Despite the attempts to protect the rhabdo-sphincter by the urethral warming device and continuously monitoring the temperature in the vicinity of the sphincter, the incidence of the incontinence following the procedure may be as high as 5% [49].
- *Urethral sloughing*. Due to the universal use of the urethral warming device in new cryo-systems, this complication is virtually not seen in the late series [50].

Oncological Outcomes

As the prostate remains in situ after the procedure, there is no universally accepted definition of biochemical failure in the case of cryotherapy. The urethra is preserved together with periurethral prostatic tissue, which may be the source of the PSA production.

According to the different series, it appears that prostate cryoablation can result in 5 year DFS of 36-92% [49, 51-55], using different definitions of failure. The reported incidence of the post-treatment negative biopsy is as high as 87-92.3% [49, 56], favorably compared with the results of external beam radiation therapy: 71.1% [56].

High Intensity Focused Ultrasound (HIFU)

Treatment Principles

HIFU is a technique that employs focused ultra-sound waves both to generate areas of extreme heat (high energy transducer) and to image the prostate gland (low energy transducer). The specially designed rectal probe is placed in a similar fashion to a TRUS probe and has a cooling balloon around it in order to prevent an injury to rectal wall.

The individual ultrasound waves produced radially by the device do not cause significant heating and tissue destruction, thus sparing rectal mucosa. However, at the focal point where all of the ultrasound waves converge or are focused, temperatures can reach well in excess of 70 degrees Celsius. These high temperatures result in the tissue essentially being cooked with subsequent coagulative necrosis. Currently, there are two commercially available HIFU units in clinical use.

Table 1. Technical characteristics of HIFU Devices

Characteristics	Sonoblate 500®	Ablatherm TM®
Patient Position	Lithotomy	Right Lateral Decubitus
Software	Semi-automated	Automated
Power	Manually Adjusted	Predetermined Settings: Primary, Salvage or Re-HIFU
Temperature Range	80-98°C	>85°C
Ablation Volume	21-47 mm	29-36 mm
Treatment Frequency	4 MHz	3 MHz
Focal Point	30-50mm	45mm
Treatment Algorithm	One	Three
Unit	Portable	Integrated table

The Ablatherm TM® device (EDAP-TMS SA, Vaulx-en Velin, France) and the Sonoblate 500® (Focus Surgery Inc, Indianapolis, IN USA. Both devices are approved for commercial use in the European Union, Canada, Russia and South Korea [57], but have not received FDA approval in the United States. It is important to realize that these two devices have specific differences with regards to limitations on patient selection, as well as technical differences in intra-operative monitoring [58, 59]. Table 1 shows the technical characteristics of HIFU devices commercially available.

Indications and Contraindications

Indications are identical to cryotherapy. The main limitation is the prostate size: patients with the glands larger than 40 ml are not advised to choose this approach [60].

The presence of significant calcification within the prostate gland is also a contraindication to the treatment as this leads to interference with the acoustic waves and can result in undertreated areas anterior to the calcification and excessive reflected heat generated posterior to it.

Rectal pathology is a relative contraindication to HIFU given the large size of the probe and the risk of fistula formation with the combination of probe trauma and treatment.

Procedure

After induction of a general or regional anesthesia the patient is placed in lithotomy position and a supra-pubic catheter is inserted. The special cradle is mounted to the table that will hold the HIFU probe. The cooling balloon is filled with water and the planning of the treatment is performed using the imaging US both in sagittal and coronal planes, followed by the systematic treatment of the gland.

Postoperative Management

The patient can be discharged on the same day or on the day following the surgery. The supra-pubic catheter is removed after the voiding trial 10-14 days later.

Complications

The incidence of complications has decreased with the advance of the techniques being used and in the recent series the erectile dysfunction is reported appear in 20-77% and urinary incontinence of any degree in 8.1% [57]. Urinary retention occurs in less than 9% of the patients and rectal fistula formation is reported not to exceed 1% [57].

Oncological Outcomes

No randomized clinical trials have been published yet comparing HIFU with other accepted approached to treat prostate cancer. In the last systematic review, Lukka et al [57] report negative biopsy rates between 35 to 95.1% in 21 series. The reported five-year DFS ranges from 55-95% in five series (measured either as three consecutive PSA rises after a nadir or as the initiation of salvage therapy) [57].

Prostate Surgery for Benign Disease

Patients who require intervention due to the benign prostate enlargement due to symptomatic voiding dysfunction and not well controlled with medical treatment may choose from a very wide range of procedures that take advantage of almost any kind of energy that humankind has discovered [61].

The list includes laser technology, electromagnetic radiation of different wave lengths including radiofrequency and microwave; electricity and simply stenting the prostatic urethra. Here we will briefly describe most of these techniques.

The most common and time honored procedure for treatment of BPH is trans-urethral resection of prostate (TURP) [62].

The indications for the operation include worsening of the lower urinary tract symptoms beyond the level the patient can bear with maximal medical treatment or individuals unable or unwilling to take medications for voiding dysfunction. In addition, patients who suffer from refractory urinary retention, recurrent urinary tract infections (UTI) due to obstructing prostate, refractory macrohematuria from the prostate, bladder calculi and obstructive uropathy secondary to BPH are indications to perform TURP.

The contraindications to the procedure are few and include significant comorbidities that pose significant risk of anesthesia or surgery and patients who are very unlikely to void spontaneously even after TURP (e.g. atonic neurogenic bladder).

Patients with proven bacteriuria and indwelling urinary catheters may benefit from preoperative antibiotic prophylaxis in order to prevent postoperative septicemia [63]. There is no need in other special preparation. After inducing regional or general anesthesia the patient is placed in dorsal lithotomy position and the genital area is prepped with antiseptic solution.

This procedure, like all endoscopic procedures, requires continuous irrigation with fluid during its performance. Unfortunately, hypotonic solutions like sterile water gain quick access to the blood stream through open blood vessels and cause hemolysis.

To overcome this life-threatening complication urologists use non-hemolitic solutions (1.5% glycine, mannitol etc). Although these solutions do not cause hemolysis, upon excessive absorption into systemic circulation they can still bring the patient to severe hyponatremia with resultant brain edema (the so called TURP syndrome).

The procedure starts with inserting transurethral resectoscope and is performed using either mono-polar or bi-polar electro-cautery. The main advantage in using the bipolar cautery is in that it allows irrigating the prostate with physiologic solution containing NaCl, which is not possible with monopolar cauterization. The use of physiologic solution prevents development of TURP syndrome.

The central portion of the obstructing prostate is removed stepwise by specially designed loop electrode using the cutting setting. The care is taken not to injure the external urinary rhabdosphincter which is close to the prostate apex and not to perforate the prostate capsule.

The chips of the prostate tissue are then irrigated out of the bladder, all bleeding vessels are coagulated and the patient is left with large bore indwelling urethral catheter for irrigation for 24 to 72 hours. If necessary, the urinary bladder stones can be fragmented and removed with the same approach during the procedure.

Intra-Operative Complications

- *Excessive bleeding:* The bleeding is best managed by prevention, i.e. prompt cauterizing large vessels that are prone to bleed because delay in doing so may cause obscured vision and they are difficult to found later.

- *TURP syndrome:* TURP syndrome is now a rare complication, but is a profound, acute hyponatremia secondary to hemodilution by the irrigation solution during a TURP. The solution gains access to the circulation through open veins in the operation field and through perforations in the prostate capsule. If not recognized, this hyponatremia can result in life-threatening cerebral edema. The condition should be prospectively sought for if the operation takes more than 1 hour, if there is an excessive bleeding and in patients with large (more than 100 ml) prostates. In addition, when the brain edema develops the patient under regional anesthesia may complain on blurred vision, diplopia and nausea. In the case of general anesthesia, signs of Cushing's can be present: elevated systemic blood pressure with reflex bradycardia secondary to elevated intra-cranial pressure. Expeditious treatment can virtually cure the patient without leaving any sequel. The surgeon has to terminate the procedure immediately, stopping to infuse more solution into the blood, switching the irrigation solution to normal saline and also to administer NaCl 0.9% intravenously. In rare severe cases there is a need to infuse hypertonic saline.
- *Prostate capsule perforation:* If the perforation of the prostate capsule is recognized during the resection, the procedure should be stopped, as large amount of non-salt containing solution will gain access to the circulation, precipitating the TURP syndrome.
- *Ureteral orifice injury:* Both ureteral orifices should be identified prior to resection in order to spare them from suffering from cautery associated injury. It may be sometimes difficult to accomplish in patients with large median lobes and with severely trabeculated bladders [64]. If there is suspicion of such an injury, the patient should be followed for urine output and flank pain postoperatively. The transient mild hydronephrosis may be caused by edema in the trigonal area and usually needs no treatment.
- *Intraoperative priapism:* It is very rare complication that may interfere with the resection of the prostate. It is taken care of with intracavernosal injection of phenylephrine 200 μg/ml in normal saline.

Post-Operative Complications

- *Urinary incontinence:* The urinary rhabdosphincter of membranous urethra is situated distal to the prostate apex and is prone to the thermal injury during a TURP. Thus, it is prudent to avoid using excessive energy at the apex area. Nonetheless, the incidence of longstanding urinary stress incontinence secondary to TURP does not exceed 5% in recent series [64].
- *Retrograde ejaculation:* This is actually not side effect, but a sequela of the surgery and is reported by the majority of the patients [64], but may be prevented by sparing the tissue around the *verumontanum.*
- *Impotence:* It is still very much controversial whether the TURP can directly cause erectile dysfunction [65], but it is generally accepted that between five to 10% of patients report worsening of erectile function following the transurethral surgery.In patients with larger than 100 gram prostates, the TURP may be quite challenging, especially when using the monopolar cautery. This approach is reported to be associated with higher incidence of postoperative hyponatremia [66]. The open approach is reserved to the patients with large prostates, but experienced surgeons can resect transurethrally prostates as large as 200 grams without increase in morbidity. Nonetheless, the open approach to benign prostate disease is reserved to prostates larger than 100 grams. The procedure can be performed through either suprapubic [67] or retropubic [68] approach. The advantage of suprapubic method is in direct access to the bladder, so the additional pathology (e.g. bladder diverticulae and calculi) may be addressed. On the other hand, the benefits of the retropubic surgery are in (i) direct visualization and exposure of the prostate and the prostate fossa, (ii) and minimal or no trauma to the bladder. The incidence of complications after open surgery is comparable to the transurethral approach, with obvious exclusion of post-operative hyponatremia. The long-term results in terms of voiding function are comparable to that of minimally invasive techniques [69].

Other Minimally Invasive Techniques for the Treatment of BPH

Holmium Laser Enucleation of the Prostate (HoLEP)

Different laser technologies have been introduced to replace the TURP, the most prevalent being HoLEP and PVP. HoLEP uses wavelength of

2140nm with pulse duration of 350ms and with this properties causes vaporization and coagulation of the prostate tissue, with thermal damage limited only to 0.5-1mm in depth [70], but requires direct contact with the tissue. Upon activation it acts as a precise knife, allowing cutting, dissecting and enucleating the prostate. During the procedure the prostate is gradually dissected from its capsule and pushed into the urinary bladder, creating the defect similar to TURP. The resected prostate is then morcellated and removed by irrigation.

Photoselective Vaporization of the Prostate (PVP)

Here the laser beam is passed through KTP crystal (kalium-titanyl-phosphate), resulting in wavelength of 1064 to 532nm (GreenLight laser). With these properties the laser energy is absorbed selectively by hemoglobin which acts as a natural chromophore, thus causing rapid vaporization of the tissue with only 1mm rim of coagulation [70]. Different from the HoLEP, it is a side firing laser. This treatment can be performed even on the patients on the full anticoagulant therapy.

Both HoLEP and PVP have been shown as promising alternatives to the TURP both in terms of functional results and in complications profile [70].

Transurethral Microwave Therapy (TUMT)

In this technique, the specially designed catheter with microwave antenna is inserted into the bladder, emitting radio waves.

The temperature in the prostate reaches above 70ºC, causing coagulation and apoptosis.

This procedure can be performed in patients with multiple comorbidities, in whom the TURP may be contraindicated. On the other hand, the procedure is not as effective as TURP when objective signs of urinary obstruction are measured [71].

Transurethral Needle Ablation of the Prostate (TUNA)

With this approach the special catheter with two adjustable needles is used, which can be deployed into the prostate tissue with high precision.

The catheter is connected to the generator of a monopolar radio-frequency signal of 490 kHz. The resulting necrotic tissue is later sloughed and voided.

Conclusion

There is a great diversity of different modalities that are in clinical use treating both malignant and benign prostate pathology. Most of them employ the latest advances in many technological fields, but the time honored approaches like the open radical prostatectomy and the TURP are still in wide use and all clinical trials studying new technologies refer to them as to the "gold standard" treatments.

References

[1] Fenter TC, Naslund MJ, Shah MB, Eaddy MT, Black L. The cost of treating the 10 most prevalent diseases in men 50 years of age or older. *Am. J. Manag. Care*. 2006 Mar; 12(4 Suppl):S90-8.

[2] Jemal A, Siegel R, Xu J, Ward E. Cancer statistics, 2010. *CA Cancer J. Clin.*, 2010 Sep-Oct; 60(5):277-300.

[3] Ferlay J, Parkin DM, Steliarova-Foucher E. Estimates of cancer incidence and mortality in Europe in 2008. *Eur. J Cancer*, Mar; 46(4):765-81.

[4] Mohler J, Bahnson RR, Boston B, Busby JE, D'Amico A, Eastham JA, et al. NCCN clinical practice guidelines in oncology: prostate cancer. *J. Natl. Compr. Canc. Netw.*, 2010 Feb; 8(2):162-200.

[5] Young HH. The early diagnosis and radical cure of carcinoma of the prostate. Being a study of 40 cases and presentation of a radical operation which was carried out in four cases. 1905. *J. Urol.*, 2002 Sep; 168(3):914-21.

[6] Walsh PC, Lepor H, Eggleston JC. Radical prostatectomy with preservation of sexual function: anatomical and pathological considerations. *Prostate*, 1983; 4(5):473-85.

[7] Chelsky MJ, Schnall MD, Seidmon EJ, Pollack HM. Use of endorectal surface coil magnetic resonance imaging for local staging of prostate cancer. *J. Urol.*, 1993 Aug; 150(2 Pt 1):391-5.

[8] Wolf JS, Jr., Bennett CJ, Dmochowski RR, Hollenbeck BK, Pearle MS, Schaeffer AJ. Best practice policy statement on urologic surgery antimicrobial prophylaxis. *J. Urol.*, 2008 Apr; 179(4):1379-90.

[9] Finley DS, Deane L, Rodriguez E, Vallone J, Deshmukh S, Skarecky D, et al. Anatomic excision of anterior prostatic fat at radical

prostatectomy: implications for pathologic upstaging. *Urology*, 2007 Nov; 70(5):1000-3.

[10] Ong AM, Su LM, Varkarakis I, Inagaki T, Link RE, Bhayani SB, et al. Nerve sparing radical prostatectomy: effects of hemostatic energy sources on the recovery of cavernous nerve function in a canine model. *J. Urol.*, 2004 Oct; 172(4 Pt 1):1318-22.

[11] Forster JA, Palit V, Myatt A, Hadi S, Bryan NP. Technical description and outcomes of a continuous anastomosis in open radical prostatectomy. *BJU Int.*, 2009 Oct; 104(7):929-33.

[12] Borland RN, Walsh PC. The management of rectal injury during radical retropubic prostatectomy. *J Urol.*, 1992 Mar; 147(3 Pt 2):905-7.

[13] Spaliviero M, Steinberg AP, Kaouk JH, Desai MM, Hammert WC, Gill IS. Laparoscopic injury and repair of obturator nerve during radical prostatectomy. *Urology*, 2004 Nov; 64(5):1030.

[14] Hedican SP, Walsh PC. Postoperative bleeding following radical retropubic prostatectomy. *J. Urol.*, 1994 Oct; 152(4):1181-3.

[15] Alemozaffar M, Regan MM, Cooperberg MR, Wei JT, Michalski JM, Sandler HM, et al. Prediction of erectile function following treatment for prostate cancer. *JAMA*, 2011 Sep 21; 306(11):1205-14.

[16] Sanda MG, Dunn RL, Michalski J, Sandler HM, Northouse L, Hembroff L, et al. Quality of life and satisfaction with outcome among prostate-cancer survivors. *N. Engl. J. Med.*, 2008 Mar 20; 358(12):1250-61.

[17] Mulhall JP, Bella AJ, Briganti A, McCullough A, Brock G. Erectile function rehabilitation in the radical prostatectomy patient. *J. Sex Med.*, 2010 Apr; 7(4 Pt 2):1687-98.

[18] Walsh PC, Marschke P, Ricker D, Burnett AL. Patient-reported urinary continence and sexual function after anatomic radical prostatectomy. *Urology*, 2000 Jan; 55(1):58-61.

[19] Breyer BN, Davis CB, Cowan JE, Kane CJ, Carroll PR. Incidence of bladder neck contracture after robot-assisted laparoscopic and open radical prostatectomy. *BJU Int.*, 2010 Dec; 106(11):1734-8.

[20] Cookson MS, Aus G, Burnett AL, Canby-Hagino ED, D'Amico AV, Dmochowski RR, et al. Variation in the definition of biochemical recurrence in patients treated for localized prostate cancer: the American Urological Association Prostate Guidelines for Localized Prostate Cancer Update Panel report and recommendations for a standard in the reporting of surgical outcomes. *J. Urol.*, 2007 Feb; 177(2):540-5.

[21] Gillitzer R, Melchior SW, Hampel C, Pahernik S, Fichtner J, Thuroff JW. Surgical atlas: Radical perineal prostatectomy. *BJU Int.*, 2004 Feb; 93(3):427-55.

[22] Walsh PC, Donker PJ. Impotence following radical prostatectomy: insight into etiology and prevention. *J. Urol.*, 1982 Sep; 128(3):492-7.

[23] Raboy A, Adler H, Albert P. Extraperitoneal endoscopic pelvic lymph node dissection: a review of 125 patients. *J. Urol.*, 1997 Dec; 158(6):2202-4; discussion 4-5.

[24] Weldon V. Radical perineal prostatectomy. In: Crawford E, Das, S, editor. Current Genitourinary Cancer Surgery. 2nd ed. Baltimore: *Williams and Wilkins*; 1997. p. 258-87.

[25] Shay BF, Schmidt JD, Thomas R, Monga M. Urology practice patterns after residency training in radical perineal prostatectomy. *Urology*, 2002 Nov; 60(5):766-9.

[26] Price DT, Vieweg J, Roland F, Coetzee L, Spalding T, Iselin C, et al. Transient lower extremity neurapraxia associated with radical perineal prostatectomy: a complication of the exaggerated lithotomy position. *J. Urol.*, 1998 Oct; 160(4):1376-8.

[27] Lance RS, Freidrichs PA, Kane C, Powell CR, Pulos E, Moul JW, et al. A comparison of radical retropubic with perineal prostatectomy for localized prostate cancer within the Uniformed Services Urology Research Group. *BJU Int.*, 2001 Jan; 87(1):61-5.

[28] Salomon L, Levrel O, de la Taille A, Anastasiadis AG, Saint F, Zaki S, et al. Radical prostatectomy by the retropubic, perineal and laparoscopic approach: 12 years of experience in one center. *Eur. Urol.*, 2002 Aug; 42(2):104-10; discussion 10-1.

[29] May M, Dorst M, May J, Hoschke B, Fahlenkamp D, Vogler H, et al. Radical retropubic vs. radical perineal prostatectomy: a comparison of relative benefits in four urban hospitals. *Urol. Nurs.*, 2007 Dec; 27(6):519-26.

[30] Prasad SM, Gu X, Lavelle R, Lipsitz SR, Hu JC. Comparative effectiveness of perineal versus retropubic and minimally invasive radical prostatectomy. *J. Urol.*, 2010 Jan; 185(1):111-5.

[31] Zuo W, Hiraoka Y. Clinical comparative evaluation of radical retropubic and perineal prostatectomy approaches for prostate cancer. *Hinyokika Kiyo*, 2003 Jan; 49(1):11-6.

[32] Schuessler WW, Schulam PG, Clayman RV, Kavoussi LR. Laparoscopic radical prostatectomy: initial short-term experience. *Urology*, 1997 Dec; 50(6):854-7.

[33] Jacob F, Salomon L, Hoznek A, Bellot J, Antiphon P, Chopin DK, et al. Laparoscopic radical prostatectomy: preliminary results. *Eur. Urol.*, 2000 May; 37(5):615-20.

[34] Guillonneau B, Vallancien G. Laparoscopic radical prostatectomy: the Montsouris technique. *J. Urol.*, 2000 Jun; 163(6):1643-9.

[35] Abbou CC, Hoznek A, Salomon L, Olsson LE, Lobontiu A, Saint F, et al. Laparoscopic radical prostatectomy with a remote controlled robot. *J. Urol.*, 2001 Jun; 165(6 Pt 1):1964-6.

[36] Binder J, Kramer W. Robotically-assisted laparoscopic radical prostatectomy. *BJU Int.*, 2001 Mar; 87(4):408-10.

[37] Bolenz C, Gupta A, Hotze T, Ho R, Cadeddu JA, Roehrborn CG, et al. Cost comparison of robotic, laparoscopic, and open radical prostatectomy for prostate cancer. *Eur. Urol.*, Mar; 57(3):453-8.

[38] Finkelstein J, Eckersberger E, Sadri H, Taneja SS, Lepor H, Djavan B. Open Versus Laparoscopic Versus Robot-Assisted Laparoscopic Prostatectomy: The European and US Experience. *Rev. Urol.*, 2010 Winter; 12(1):35-43.

[39] Briganti A, Gallina A, Suardi N, Capitanio U, Tutolo M, Bianchi M, et al. Predicting erectile function recovery after bilateral nerve sparing radical prostatectomy: a proposal of a novel preoperative risk stratification. *J. Sex Med.*, Jul; 7(7):2521-31.

[40] Chauhan S, Coelho RF, Rocco B, Palmer KJ, Orvieto MA, Patel VR. Techniques of nerve-sparing and potency outcomes following robot-assisted laparoscopic prostatectomy. *Int. Braz. J. Urol.*, 2010 May-Jun; 36(3):259-72.

[41] Frota R, Turna B, Barros R, Gill IS. Comparison of radical prostatectomy techniques: open, laparoscopic and robotic assisted. *Int. Braz. J. Urol.*, 2008 May-Jun; 34(3):259-68; discussion 68-9.

[42] Patel VR, Coelho RF, Rocco B, Orvieto M, Sivaraman A, Palmer KJ, et al. Positive surgical margins after robotic assisted radical prostatectomy: a multi-institutional study. *J. Urol.*, 2011 Aug; 186(2):511-6.

[43] Coelho RF, Rocco B, Patel MB, Orvieto MA, Chauhan S, Ficarra V, et al. Retropubic, laparoscopic, and robot-assisted radical prostatectomy: a critical review of outcomes reported by high-volume centers. *J. Endourol.*, 2010 Dec; 24(12):2003-15.

[44] Cooper IS, Hirose T. Application of cryogenic surgery to resection of parenchymal organs. *N. Engl. J. Med.*, 1966 Jan 6; 274(1):15-8.

[45] Larson TR, Rrobertson DW, Corica A, Bostwick DG. In vivo interstitial temperature mapping of the human prostate during cryosurgery with

correlation to histopathologic outcomes. *Urology*, 2000 Apr; 55(4): 547-52.

[46] Williams AK, Martinez CH, Lu C, Ng CK, Pautler SE, Chin JL. Disease-free survival following salvage cryotherapy for biopsy-proven radio-recurrent prostate cancer. *Eur. Urol.*, 2011 Sep; 60(3):405-10.

[47] Babaian RJ, Donnelly B, Bahn D, Baust JG, Dineen M, Ellis D, et al. Best practice statement on cryosurgery for the treatment of localized prostate cancer. *J. Urol.*, 2008 Nov; 180(5):1993-2004.

[48] Prepelica KL, Okeke Z, Murphy A, Katz AE. Cryosurgical ablation of the prostate: high risk patient outcomes. *Cancer*, 2005 Apr 15; 103(8):1625-30.

[49] Bahn DK, Lee F, Badalament R, Kumar A, Greski J, Chernick M. Targeted cryoablation of the prostate: 7-year outcomes in the primary treatment of prostate cancer. *Urology*, 2002 Aug; 60(2 Suppl 1):3-11.

[50] De La Taille A, Benson MC, Bagiella E, Burchardt M, Shabsigh A, Olsson CA, et al. Cryoablation for clinically localized prostate cancer using an argon-based system: complication rates and biochemical recurrence. *BJU Int.*, 2000 Feb; 85(3):281-6.

[51] Long JP, Fallick ML, LaRock DR, Rand W. Preliminary outcomes following cryosurgical ablation of the prostate in patients with clinically localized prostate carcinoma. *J. Urol.*, 1998 Feb; 159(2):477-84.

[52] Han KR, Cohen JK, Miller RJ, Pantuck AJ, Freitas DG, Cuevas CA, et al. Treatment of organ confined prostate cancer with third generation cryosurgery: preliminary multicenter experience. *J Urol.*, 2003 Oct; 170(4 Pt 1):1126-30.

[53] Levy DA, Pisters LL, Jones JS. Primary cryoablation nadir prostate specific antigen and biochemical failure. *J. Urol.*, 2009 Sep; 182(3): 931-7.

[54] Jones JS, Rewcastle JC, Donnelly BJ, Lugnani FM, Pisters LL, Katz AE. Whole gland primary prostate cryoablation: initial results from the cryo on-line data registry. *J. Urol.*, 2008 Aug; 180(2):554-8.

[55] Hubosky SG, Fabrizio MD, Schellhammer PF, Barone BB, Tepera CM, Given RW. Single center experience with third-generation cryosurgery for management of organ-confined prostate cancer: critical evaluation of short-term outcomes, complications, and patient quality of life. *J. Endourol.*, 2007 Dec; 21(12):1521-31.

[56] Donnelly BJ, Saliken JC, Brasher PM, Ernst SD, Rewcastle JC, Lau H, et al. A randomized trial of external beam radiotherapy versus

cryoablation in patients with localized prostate cancer. *Cancer*, 2010 Jan 15; 116(2):323-30.

[57] Lukka H, Waldron T, Chin J, Mayhew L, Warde P, Winquist E, et al. High-intensity focused ultrasound for prostate cancer: a systematic review. *Clin. Oncol.*, (R Coll Radiol). 2010 Mar; 23(2):117-27.

[58] Chaussy C, Thuroff S, Rebillard X, Gelet A. Technology insight: High-intensity focused ultrasound for urologic cancers. *Nat. Clin. Pract. Urol.*, 2005 Apr; 2(4):191-8.

[59] Uchida T, Sanghvi NT, Gardner TA, Koch MO, Ishii D, Minei S, et al. Transrectal high-intensity focused ultrasound for treatment of patients with stage T1b-2n0m0 localized prostate cancer: a preliminary report. *Urology*, 2002 Mar; 59(3):394-8; discussion 8-9.

[60] Gelet A, Chapelon JY, Bouvier R, Rouviere O, Lyonnet D, Dubernard JM. Transrectal high intensity focused ultrasound for the treatment of localized prostate cancer: factors influencing the outcome. *Eur. Urol.*, 2001 Aug; 40(2):124-9.

[61] Burke N, Whelan JP, Goeree L, Hopkins RB, Campbell K, Goeree R, et al. Systematic review and meta-analysis of transurethral resection of the prostate versus minimally invasive procedures for the treatment of benign prostatic obstruction. *Urology*, 2010 May; 75(5):1015-22.

[62] Smith RD, Patel A. Transurethral resection of the prostate revisited and updated. *Curr. Opin. Urol.*, 2011 Jan; 21(1):36-41.

[63] Qiang W, Jianchen W, MacDonald R, Monga M, Wilt TJ. Antibiotic prophylaxis for transurethral prostatic resection in men with preoperative urine containing less than 100,000 bacteria per ml: a systematic review. *J. Urol.*, 2005 Apr; 173(4):1175-81.

[64] Rassweiler J, Teber D, Kuntz R, Hofmann R. Complications of transurethral resection of the prostate (TURP)--incidence, management, and prevention. *Eur. Urol.*, 2006 Nov; 50(5):969-79; discussion 80.

[65] Lynch MJ. Transurethral resection of the prostate stands accused of causing impotence in patients: should it be found culpable? *BJU Int.*, 2010 Sep; 106(5):614-9.

[66] Kwon JS, Lee JW, Lee SW, Choi HY, Moon HS. Comparison of effectiveness of monopolar and bipolar transurethral resection of the prostate and open prostatectomy in large benign prostatic hyperplasia. *Korean J. Urol.*, 2011 Apr; 52(4):269-73.

[67] Freyer PJ. Total Enucleation of the Prostate: A Further Series of 550 Cases of the Operation. *Br. Med. J.*, 1919 Feb 1; 1(3031):121-0 2.

[68] Millin T. Retropubic prostatectomy; a new extravesical technique; report of 20 cases. *Lancet*, 1945 Dec 1; 2(6380):693-6.

[69] Alivizatos G, Skolarikos A, Chalikopoulos D, Papachristou C, Sopilidis O, Dellis A, et al. Transurethral photoselective vaporization versus transvesical open enucleation for prostatic adenomas >80ml: 12-mo results of a randomized prospective study. *Eur. Urol.*, 2008 Aug; 54(2):427-37.

[70] Gravas S, Bachmann A, Reich O, Roehrborn CG, Gilling PJ, De La Rosette J. Critical review of lasers in benign prostatic hyperplasia (BPH). *BJU Int.*, 2011 Apr; 107(7):1030-43.

[71] Frieben RW, Lin HC, Hinh PP, Berardinelli F, Canfield SE, Wang R. The impact of minimally invasive surgeries for the treatment of symptomatic benign prostatic hyperplasia on male sexual function: a systematic review. *Asian. J. Androl.*, 2010 Jul; 12(4):500-8.

In: Prostatectomies
Editors: H. Alvelos and Y. Izidoro
ISBN: 978-1- 62081-077-4
© 2012 Nova Science Publishers, Inc.

Chapter II

Suprapubic Prostatectomy for Benign Prostatic Hyperplasia: Aspects of Evolution of Hemostatic Methods to Present Time

***Chukwudi O. Okorie*[1] *and Louis L. Pisters*[2]**
[1]Pan African Academy of Christian Surgeons at Tenwek Hospital, Bomet, Kenya
[2]University of Texas M.D. Anderson Cancer Center, Dept. of Urology, Holcombe Blvd., Houston, Texas, US

Abstract

Suprapubic prostatectomy for benign prostatic hyperplasia (BPH) remains a viable option in the surgical treatment of BPH for the adequately selected patients and is the predominant method of surgical treatment of BPH in the developing world. One of the discouraging aspects of suprapubic prostatectomy is the frequent and significant hemorrhage that can be encountered. Controlling hemorrhage after suprapubic prostatectomy has always been a point of research from the time this method of surgery was developed. At present time it can be said that controlling hemostasis is one of the key factors to a safe and successful outcome of suprapubic prostatectomy. The difficulties encountered over the years in achieving good hemostasis has continued to frustrate many urologists involved in doing this surgery. In this paper we give a brief history of methods previously used to achieve hemostasis during suprapubic prostatectomy and then highlight our method of hemostasis which in our experience has been very effective in controlling bleeding during suprapubic prostatectomy.

1. Introduction

Suprapubic prostatectomy remains a viable option in the surgical treatment of benign prostatic hyperplasia (BPH) and is the most effective surgical method for relieving symptoms of obstructive urination caused by benign prostatic hyperplasia with a low re-treatment rate [1]. In contemporary practice, indications for suprapubic prostatectomy include presence of large BPH, absence of necessary technology for alternative procedures especially in low resource economies, presence of concomitant pathological conditions like stones, bladder diverticula and for patients for whom positioning for endoscopic procedure may not be feasible for example in patients with pelvic/hip joint deformities. Furthermore, in many low resource economies, many of the BPH surgery are still done by general surgeons and even general medical practitioners and majority of these doctors find the suprapubic approach easier to learn compared to the retropubic approach. Results of contemporary studies do show that suprapubic prostatectomy is a very effective surgical procedure for BPH with both good short term and long term outcome [2,3,4,5,6,7,8]. Improvement in hemostasis during suprapubic prostatectomy has been one of the key factors in reducing mortality that was high in the early years of this surgery compared to contemporary series. In the early years of this surgical method, one of the leading causes of death was hemorrhage [9]. Nanninga JB and O'Conor VJ [9] in their review of four series of suprapubic prostatectromy reported a decrease in mortality from 8.5% to 1.4% and attributed this decline in mortality to improvement in hemostatsis among other contributing factors . With significant improvement in surgical technique of suprapubic prostatectomy and drastic reduction in the mortality, the need for blood transfusion has now become the key factor in determining adequacy of hemostasis during above surgery. In the series of suprapubic prosataectomy reported by Nanninga JB and O'Conor VJ [9] from 1953 to 1961, there were no fatalities attributed to hemorrhage however the blood transfusion rate was 31%. In more recent publications, the transfusion rate has remained variable and most likely reflects the technique and experience of the involved surgeon. In many hands the transfusion rate has significantly decreased [3,7] and even reaching the zero percent mark [6,10,11] while in others the transfusion rate has remained high with little or no difference from series reported many decades ago [12,13]. The search for the perfect method of hemostasis has been long and creative to say the least and has ranged from packing of the prostatic fossa to different forms of suture application to the bladder neck and prostatic cavity. The results of these different approaches have been mixed ranging from good to inadequate haemostatic control with major complications including post-operative bladder neck stenosis, urinary fistulae, and the need to re-operate due to clot retention, bladder rupture, or in a delayed manner, stricture of the lower urinary tract. The mixed results with modified surgical techniques have continued to frustrate many urologists and other surgeons or physicians interested in doing this surgery. Effective hemostasis with minimal or no associated complications therefore remains one of the key goals of any suprapubic prostatectomy. In this paper, we will look at evolution of hemostatic methods that had led to most of the contemporary practices with latter emphasis on the author's technique.

2. Methods of Hemostasis for Suprapubic Prostatectomy

2.1. Packing of Cavities

One of the earliest attempts at achieving haemostasis during suprapubic prostatectomy was through packing of cavities: initially the bladder cavity was packed and later the prostatic fossa became the main focus of packing. The earliest surgeons that used packing of the bladder cavity included Belfield and McGill [14], it has to be stated however that these early surgeons [15,16] until the era of Fuller [17], accomplished partial removal of the hyperplastic prostatic tissue. Packing of the prostatic fossa soon became the preferred technique by most surgeons as a better method of stopping and preventing hemorrhage during suprapubic prostatectomy. Plain Gauze has been the material commonly used for the packing. Other materials used included oxidized cellulose gauze [18] and gel foam pack [19]. To further enhance the effectiveness of the packing method, some surgeons added adrenalin to the plain gauze [20]. The reported advantage of the oxidized cellulose gauze was the possibility of complete absorption into the tissues and as such no need for later removal however it was associated with calculus formation that in the hands of Baker and Graf [21] needed cystoscopic removal. The mechanism of action of gauze packing can be attributed to mechanical pressure on the bleeding surfaces and also to inducement of clotting by the gauze material used for the packing. Generally, packing has been associated with mixed success in controlling hemorrhage with not uncommon need to periodically re-pack few hours following surgery due to persistent bleeding. Even in cases were packing helped achieve control of hemostasis, periodic drainage of urine to the exterior through the exit site, later removal of the gauze pack that can be painful and can also provoke re-bleeding due to dislodgement of the already formed clot on the prostatic fossa further decreased the appeal of this method. To avoid pain and also to be ready for possible re-packing, many urologists removed the gauze pack in the operating room with the use of anesthesia and as such subjecting involved patients to another trip to the operating room [22]. Some contemporary authors have however reported more successful outcome of prostatic fossa packing with lower complication rates [11,13].

2.2. Hemostatic Bags

Hemostatic bags can be considered as having evolved from the concept of packing the prostatic fossa. The earliest innovation in this technique was probably by Briggs and not Hagner who has been generally credited with developing the first of these bags [22]. In this technique, special inflatable bags were used to apply pressure to the bleeding vessels in the prostatic fossa. While these bags were reported to have achieved some level of success in controlling hemostasis, they were also reported to frequently slip out of the prostatic fossa where they were subsequently of little use leading to a series of creative innovations to hold the hemostatic bags in place in the prostatic cavity [22]. The development of the Foley hemostatic catheter [23] can be seen as the final innovation of these many and various types of hemostatic bags. The Foley 'hemostatic' catheter was initially intended for use after transurethral resection of the prostate but was then widely adopted and used after suprapubic prostatectomy [22]. Contemporary studies done using Foley catheter traction after trans-urethral resection of the prostate (TURP) has shown reduction in post TURP bleeding [24] and same can be expected after suprapubic prostatectomy. Most surgeons will have the balloon of the catheter under traction inside the bladder lumen however the preference of having the balloon of the Foley catheter inside the prostatic fossa by some surgeons during suprapubic prostatectomy can be assumed to be one the contemporary application of the concept of hemostatic bags in its original intent [2,25].

2.3. Application of Heat

Different forms of heat have been used towards achieving hemostasis after suprapubic prostatectomy. Fuller used irrigation of the bladder with hot water while McGill and Guiteras advocated irrigation of prostatic fossa with very hot water [14, 16, 26]. These practices are no longer in contemporary use however. McCarthy [27] suggested insertion of a resectoscope after suprapubic prostatectomy for coagulation of arterial bleeders. This approach did not gain wide usage probably because of its cumbersome nature. A more contemporary approach is the periodic use of electrocautery during suprapubic prostatectomy to cauterize small bleeders at the edges of the bladder neck.

2.4. Sutural Method of Hemostasis

Suturing for the purpose of effecting hemostasis can reasonably be assumed to be as old as surgery itself. With the development of suprapubic prostatectomy as a reliable surgical method of treating BPH, the efforts of generations of urologists soon became focused on developing a reliable sutural method of controlling bleeding during surgery.

With many other methods of hemostasis after suprapubic prostatectomy failing to achieve the desired goal, it was soon realized that a sutural method was a more promising alternative. This effort was greatly aided by the development of surgical instruments which among other benefits facilitated more efficient means of retraction of the bladder and visualization of the prostatic fossa to better see the location of the bleeding vessels as well as the development of better needle holders and needles that technically improved the actual process of suturing bleeders [28].

Application of stitches to bleeding points or to areas of anatomical entrance of arterial branches supplying the hyperplastic prostatatic tissues are presently the dominant method of hemostatsis during suprapubic prostatectomy. Schoonover, Lower and Harris were among the early pioneers and strong advocates of the sutural hemostasis [29, 30, 31]. There has been persistent effort among the early surgeons to place sutures at areas of the bladder neck where they thought will help achieve maximum hemostasis. Harris [31], in addition to reformation of the prostatic fossa, placed hemostatic sutures at the 5 o'clock and 7 o'clock positions of the bladder neck. Silverton RJ [28] in his surgical description of sutural hemostasis during suprapubic prostatectomy prefers to place 'U' shaped or mattress sutures more or less to include the areas between the 3 o'clock and 5 o'clock as well as between the 7 o'clock and 9 o'clock positions. Another significant development in the evolution of the sutural method of hemostasis is the concept of separating the prostatic fossa from the bladder neck.

This significant modification of sutural hemostasis has further led to a distinct line of sutural hemostasis with many reported good surgical outcomes. Lower [30] and Harris [31] were the early pioneers that described the method of separation of prostatic fossa from bladder neck using absorbable sutures as an approach to the control of hemorrhage associated with suprapubic prostatectomy. Further development of the concept of separation of the prostatic fossa from the bladder neck gave rise to the use of removable purse string suture [32]. Malamet [33] used this approach of removable suture method of separating the prostatic fossa from the bladder neck and noted significant reduction in post suprapubic prostatectomy bleeding. Other authors using the Malamet technique [34, 35, 3] documented good results and hence the Malamet technique has continued to be an option of surgical hemostasis during suprapubic prostatectomy.

Denis [36] in a further modification of the removable purse string technique additionally placed a drain in the prostatic fossa that according to the author led to retraction and tamponade of the fossa and through this combination of suturing and drain placement achieved improved hemostasis. Contemporary usage of the removable purse string technique has showed significant improvement in hemostasis, however some of the complications that has historically plagued the technique of separating the prostatic fossa from the bladder neck like bladder neck stenosis/urethral stricture, periodic need for blood transfusion, clot retention and catheter blockage has variably persisted. With this approach, there has occasionally been the need to return to operating room to remove fragments of broken purse string suture or for clot evacuation although these complications may be dependent on the surgeon or medical center [3, 7].

In contemporary practice, the most commonly recommended method of sutural hemostasis has been application of hemostatic stitches to the 5 and 7 o'clock positions of the bladder neck [37, 38]. This method of hemostasis can be effective in many of these procedures however in many other cases, significant hemorrhage and the need for blood transfusion has been a persisting problem [38] further fueling the persistent search of a more effective method of hemostasis during suprapubic prostatectomy. It will be worthwhile at this moment to look at the vascular pattern of the prostate to gain some insights on how best to approach sutural hemostasis.

3. Prostate Vascular Anatomy

In order to gain insight into the optimal approach to sutural hemostasis, it will be of great significance to review what is known on the blood supply to the prostate. Rubin Flocks [39] in his studies on the arterial blood supply to the prostate demonstrated the dual system of arterial perfusion of the BPH from the urethral arterial branches of the inferior vesical artery as well as from the capsular arteries.

According to Flocks, the urethral arterial branch provide the principal blood supply to BPH and arises from the inferior vesical artery at the 5 and 7 o'clock positions but approach the bladder neck in the 1 o'clock to 5 o'clock position and the 7 o'clock to 11 o'clock position with no vessels entering in the anterior and posterior median lines.

Clegg [40] in his study of arterial blood supply to the prostate do agree with Flocks that most vessels enter the gland between 1 and 5 o'clock position and 7 and 11 o'clock position but however disagrees on the absence of vascularization of the anterior and posterior median planes.

Bilhim T et al [41] in their study of prostatic vascularization reported that on reaching the prostatic capsule, the prostatic artery divides into several perforating branches to the gland and that the antero-lateral pedicles penetrate the gland at 2 and 10 o'clock positions while the postero-lateral pedicles penetrate the gland at 5 and 7 o'clock positions.

It does then seem that placing hemostatic stitches only at the 5 and 7 o'clock positions of the bladder neck as commonly recommended and widely practiced is not adequate in effectively controlling hemorrhage during suprapubic prostatectomy.

4. The Authors' Method of Suprapubic Prostatectomy

4.1. Pre-Operative Work-Up

In the authors practice, the transurethral resection of the prostate (TURP) is available and the main indication for suprapubic prostatectomy is related to the size of the prostate or to the presence of associated bladder pathology or stones that dictates open intervention. Preoperative evaluation is kept simplified as much as possible to include adequate history (including international prostate symptom score 'IPSS' when patients are not in retention or on catheter) and physical examination which can then lead to a more elaborate work-up depending on findings. As a minimum however, basic investigations include a hemoglobin, creatinine and urine check. Digital rectal examination also remains a basic and routine investigation while prostate specific antigen and prostate biopsy are done when deemed necessary especially on suspicious physical examination findings to exclude cases of possible prostatic cancer.

4.2. Operative Technique

It is usually helpful to fill up the bladder with normal saline before commencement of the surgery. Under spinal anesthesia as the anesthesia of choice, the skin incision for suprapubic prostatectomy can be performed either through a lower midline incision of variable length depending on surgeons preference but should be contained within the area between the umbilicus and the pubic symphysis or through a short transverse 'Pfannenstiel' incision.

The skin incision is continued through the subcutaneous tissues and fascial layers while the rectus abdominis muscles are separated in the midline. The extraperitoneal prevesical space is subsequently developed to expose the anterior bladder wall which is then opened vertically between two stay sutures. The bladder lumen is always inspected to exclude any other associated pathology that could have been missed in the pre-operative stage.

The bladder lumen may now be retracted to adequately expose the bladder neck to start finger enucleation. It is however the author's preference to enucleate bluntly and later uses retractors during sutural hemostasis.

Properly and carefully done enucleation of the hyperplastic prostatic tissue is a key and important step towards a successful outcome of suprapubic prostatectomy. Preference is routinely given to starting the enucleation process from inside the proximal urethra, carefully separating the hyperplastic prostatic tissue from the verumontanum and progressing towards the bladder neck until complete removal of the adenomatous tissues.

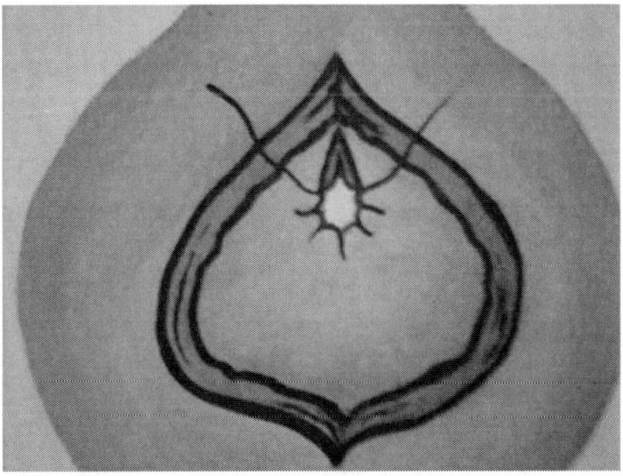

Figure 1. Running suture from 1 o'clock position to 11 o'clock position, suturing the bladder neck edge to the prostatic capsule. [Okorie CO et al: Urology 2010;75(3): 701-706.].

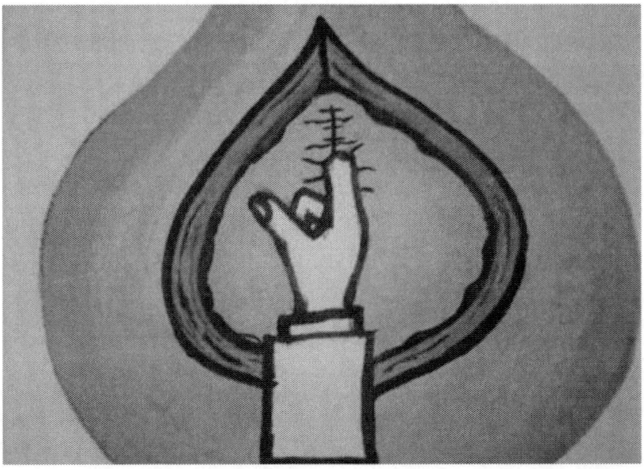

Figure 2. Bladder neck narrowed up to the diameter of the surgeon's index finger. [Okorie CO et al: Urology 2010;75(3):701-706.].

Our modified method of surgical hemostasis during suprapubic prostatectomy has some similarities with the partition method of separating the prostatic fossa from the bladder neck in the more detailed and almost circumferential suturing of the bladder neck edges to that of the prostatic fossa but significantly differs in avoiding purse string and in reconstructing the bladder neck to the diameter of the surgeon's index finger.

Hence the authors modification is based on the intent to maximize hemostatic suturing of all arterial branches that enter into the bladder neck and proximal prostatic capsule in contrast to the commonly practiced applications of stitches to the 5 and 7 o'clock positions while at same time avoiding excessive narrowing of the bladder neck that could compromise the bladder neck lumen and as such lead to prostatic fossa or bladder neck stenosis.

The modified bladder neck repair/sutural hemostasis [4,10] consists of a running suture from 1 o'clock position to 11 o'clock position, suturing the bladder neck edge to the prostatic capsule with 2-0 polyglactin suture (Figure 1) and additional interrupted sutures vertically starting from the 12 o'clock position downwards to narrow the bladder neck up to the diameter of the surgeon's index finger(Figure 2). With the index finger in the bladder neck, a 22 or 24 two-way urethral Foley catheter is inserted and guided into the bladder lumen.

The Balloon of the Foley catheter which remains in the bladder lumen is inflated to a minimum of 30ml and placed on mild traction by tying a piece of gauze to the catheter and pushing it mildly against the meatus for approximately 2 hours and additionally by taping the catheter to the thigh under moderate traction until the following morning with an adhesive strapping. In this way the catheter balloon is mildly pushed against the bladder neck augmenting hemostasis.

Anterior bladder wall defect and the rest of the incisional wound layers are closed without use of suprapubic catheters or other drains. Importantly, post-operative bladder irrigation is not needed and not utilized with this approach.

We believe our modified technique of haemostasis is easy to learn as confirmed from working with surgical residents and should hopefully go a long way to make hemorrhagic complications associated with suprapubic prostatectomy less common.

Furthermore in assisting surgical residents with different sizes of the index finger repair the bladder neck, no noticeable change in the patient's outcome has so far been noticed, hence our preliminary conclusion will be that any surgeon can safely use his or her index finger diameter to determine when to stop narrowing the bladder neck.

Acquiring this new skill of doing suprapubic prostatectomy is additionally important as the number of large prostates not amenable to TURP is on the increase especially in the western world were many patients with BPH are initially treated medically over a long period of time only to present later with large prostate glands [42].

4.3. Post-Operative Care

The need for vigilant monitoring of post suprapubic prostatectomy patients cannot be emphasized enough.

The aim of the monitoring include general follow-up of the patient's vital signs and other issues that should be addressed for any patient that have undergone any kind of major surgery. However for patients after suprapubic prostatectomy the emphasis is placed on assuring continuous functioning of the catheter and also monitoring the color of the efflux in correlation to the vital signs as a way of assessing possible ongoing hemorrhage.

Of interest was the observation that post-operative bladder drainage was periodically noted to be already clear in the operating room indicating both improved surgical hemostasis and successful prevention of reflux of blood from the prostatic fossa to the bladder lumen.

For all the patients and especially at the early stage of their post-operative recovery, it is important to ensure that there is no sign of retained clots which usually should be evident with decreased urine output and increasing suprapubic area discomfort. Should there be any doubt however; catheter function should easily be restored through aspiration and irrigation with 60cc syringe by the patient's bed side with no need to return any of these patients to the operating room.

4.4. Need for Blood Transfusion

As previously mentioned in this chapter, need for blood transfusion is presently the commonly used outcome measure in assessing the adequacy of surgical hemostasis during suprapubic prostatectomy.

Blood transfusion after suprapubic prostatectomy is still frequent and should be avoided as much as possible especially across low resource economies with frequent and persisting difficulties in blood banking.

Furthermore the high risk of transmissible infection especially the present high infection rate of HIV across many countries of the world has made any option of blood transfusion worrisome. Using our Modified technique of haemostatic control none of the patients needed blood transfusion [4,10].

4.5. Need for Post-Operative Bladder Irrigation

Post-operative bladder irrigation has been an integral part of suprapubic prostatectomy from the time of development of this surgical method and is still widely practiced [19, 37]. The aim of bladder irrigation has been to facilitate evacuation of blood from ongoing or recurrent bleeding and as such prevent clot formation and catheter blockage that could lead to a number of complications including: clot retention, bladder wall disruption, return to operating room and patient discomfort among other possible complications. Bladder irrigation demands a lot of nursing attention and in the presence of obstructed outflow; ongoing post-operative bladder irrigation can quickly lead to full bladder with significant accompanying pain and possible bladder wall disruption. Adequate hemostasis in combination with good catheter drainage should theoretically lead to reduced presence of blood in the bladder which then should lead to none or less incidences of clot formation, retention and episodes of catheter blockage.

Hence the key to elimination of bladder irrigation lies foremost with achieving effective surgical hemostasis and preventing as much as possible presence of blood in the bladder lumen through reflux of blood from the prostatic fossa as well as enhancing immediate and effective efflux of any blood that happens to get into the bladder lumen through unobstructed catheter drainage.

Apart from our modified method of bladder neck repair that improved hemostasis, other factors that helped reduce the presence of blood in the bladder included: 1. After the bladder neck is tapered and a catheter placed on mild traction, we believe that the bladder neck itself is advanced into the prostatic capsular defect and may directly compress other bleeding vessels at the prostatic capsular defect. 2. Tailoring the bladder neck to the size of an index finger and having the balloon of the Foley catheter placed inside the bladder lumen under mild traction against the bladder neck secondarily should have helped reduce back flow of blood to the bladder lumen from the prostatic fossa. The noted increased efflux of blood to the outside beside the urethral catheter with our modified surgery contrary to old series repaired traditionally indicates reduced backflow of blood into the bladder from the prostatic fossa. 3. Another additional factor that in our opinion aided successful outcome of our modified suprapubic prostatectomy without use of bladder irrigation is our use of 2- way Foley catheter instead of 3-way Foley catheter enhancing better efflux from the bladder.

This could be explained by the larger outflow lumen present in the 2-way catheter compared to 3-way catheters. Use of urethral catheters of very good quality is however emphasized as these catheters hardly collapse due to their strong walls and as such enhancing very good drainage and in cases of blockage are more easily irrigated out.

We did show in our study [4] that not only can suprapubic prostatectomy be performed safely without irrigation, but the use of irrigation can cause significant morbidity in the presence of obstructed outflow. Many other advantages of avoiding post-operative bladder irrigation include; cost and nursing workload reduction; better monitoring of urine output and increased patient comfort.

5. Issues Surrounding Adoption of New Surgical Modifications

There is no doubt that reproducibility of surgical techniques that have worked relatively well in the hands of the inventors/innovators remains a crucial factor in the outcome and general acceptability of new surgical approaches. It therefore has to be understood that modifications to surgical techniques will probably keep occurring as there is hardly any surgical approach that works or will work 100% perfect for all involved, hence success and acceptability of any modification will not only be dependent on the simplicity and effectiveness of the new modification in solving the arising problems but to a significant extent on the accurate reproducibility of the new method.

Hence a significant part of the effort to make a new method work will befall on the interested persons who should endeavor to closely reproduce the steps of the modification and also to pay needed attention to patient selection as well as to both pre-operative and post operative aspects of the surgery and as such come up with results that are very close to those of the authors if not even better with eventual aim of preventing or drastically reducing complications.

Conclusion

The search for the optimal hemostatic method during suprapubic prostatectomy has been long and creative to say the least. Each new method or modification comes with an added value to what is already known and further helps the process of achieving the desired goal of adequate hemostasis. The author's modification has strong vascular anatomic correlation and has worked very well in the author's hands and in those of many others that have reported back to the authors on their experiences with usage of this new modification. It is hoped that this modification will work for many more that will implement it and as such extend the key advantages of; avoiding blood transfusion, avoiding bladder irrigation, better monitoring of urine output, increased patient's comfort, reduced hospital cost and reduced nursing workload.

References

[1] McConnell JD, Barry MJ, Bruskewitz RC, et al. Benign prostatic hyperplasia: Diagnosis and treatment. Clinical practice guideline. AHCPR publication No 94-0582, [number 8]. Rocville, Agency for Health Care Policy and Research, Public health service, U.S. *Department of health and human services*, 1994.

[2] Tubaro A, Carter S, Hind A, Vicentini C, Maino L. A prospective study of the safety and efficacy of suprapubic transvesical prostatectomy in patients with benign prostatic hyperplasia. J Urol 2001; 166:172-176.

[3] Meier DE, Tarpley JL, Imediegwu OO, et al. The outcome of suprapubic prostatectomy: A contemporary series in the developing world. *Urology* 1995; 46:40-44.

[4] Okorie CO, Salia M, Liu P, Pisters LL. Modified suprapubic prostatectomy without irrigation is safe. *Urology* 2010;75(3):701-706.

[5] Varkarakis I, Kyriakakis Z, Delis A, Protogerou V, Deliveliotis C. Long-term results of open transvesical prostatectomy from a contemporary series of patients. *Urology* 2004; 64(2):306- 310.

[6] Lezrek M, Ameur A, Renteria JM, El Alj HA, Beddouch A. Modified Denis technique: A simple solution for maximal hemostasis in suprapubic prostatectomy. *Urology* 2003;61:951-955.

[7] Condie JD, Cutherell L Jr. Mian A. Suprapubic prostatectomy for benign prostatic hyperplasia in rural Asia: 200 consecutive cases. *Urology*. 1999;54:1012-1016.

[8] Serretta V, Morgia G, Fondacuro L et al. Open prostatectomy for benign prostatic enlargement in southern Europe in the late 1990s: A contemporary series of 1800 interventions. *Urology* 2002; 60:623-627.

[9] Nanninga JB, O'Conor VJ. Suprapubic prostatectomy: a 28 year review, 1942-1970. *International Urology and Nephrology*. 1972;4(4):377-382.

[10] Okorie CO, Pisters LL.Effect of modified suprapubic prostatectomy for benign prostatic hyperplasia on postoperative hemoglobin levels. *Can. J. Urol.* 2010 Aug;17(4): 5255-8.

[11] Mireku-Boateng AO, Jackson AG. Prostate fossa packing: a simple, quick and effective method of achieving hemostasis in suprapubic prostatectomy. *Urol. Int.* 2005;74(2):180-2.

[12] Brian Helfand, Samdeep Mouli, Raj Dedhia, Keven T. Mcvary. Management of lower urinary symptoms secondary to benign prostatic hyperplasia with open prostatectomy: Results of a contemporary series. *J. Urol.* 2006; 176:2557-2561.

[13] Bapat RD, Relekar RG, Pandit SR, Dandekar NP. Comparative study between modified Freyer's prostatectomy, classical Freyer's prostatectomy and Millin's prostatectomy. *J. Postgrad. Med.* 1991;37(1):144-147.

[14] Belfield WT. Operation on the enlarged prostate with a tabulated summary of cases. *Am. J. Med .Sci.* 1890;100:439.

[15] McGill AF. Adiscussion on the treatment of retention of urine from prostatic enlargement. *BMJ*.1889;2(Oct.19):863.

[16] Fuller E. *Diseases of the genito-urinary system*. New York. MacMillan. 1900.

[17] Fuller PJ. Six successful and successive cases of prostatectomy. *J. Cutan. Genitourin. Dis.* 1895;13:229.

[18] Fish GW. Oxidized cellulose (absorbable hemostatic gauze, cellulosic acid): its use in genitor urinary surgery. *Ibid.* 1946;56:375.

[19] Thiel DD, Petrou SP. Electroresection and open surgery. *Urol. Clin. N. Am.* 2009;36:461-470.

[20] Moullin CM. *Enlargement of the prostate*. Phildelphia. P. Blakistons Sons and Co. 1911.

[21] 21. Baker W, Graf EC. Evaluation of oxycel-bag catheters technique in suprapubic prostatectomy. *Ibid.* 1952;67:101.

[22] Herman JR, Castro L. Suprapubic prostatectomy: Some early methods of hemostasis. *Urology*. 1973;1(6):612-619.

[23] Foley FEB. A hemostatic bag catheter. *Ibid.* 1937;38:134.

[24] Walker EM, Bera S, Paiz M. Does catheter traction reduce post-transurethral resection of the prostate blood loss?. *BJU*. 1995;75: 614-617.

[25] Adam C, Hofstetler A, Deubner J, et al. Retropubic transvesical prostatectomy for significant prostatic enlargement must remain a standard part of urology training. *Scand. J. Urol. Nephrol.* 2004; 38: 472-476.

[26] Guiteras R. Urology, *the diseases of the urinary tract in men and women*, New York, D. Appleton and Co. 1912. Vol II.

[27] McCarthy JF. Discussion of Lavalle LL, and Hamm FC. Osteitis pubis. *J. Urol.* 1951;66:428.

[28] Silverton RJ. Sutural haemostasis in suprapubic prostatectomy. ANZ *Journal of Surgery.* 1934;3(3):276-83.

[29] Schoonover FS Jr. Prostatectomy: the control of hemorrhage. *Ibid.* 1925;14:57.

[30] Lower WE. Complete closure of the bladder following prostatectomy. *JAMA*. 1927;89:749- 51.

[31] Harris S. Prostatectomy with closure: Five years experience. *BJS*. 1934;21:434.

[32] De La Pena A, Alcina E. Suprapubic prostatectomy: a new technique to prevent bleeding. *J. Urol.* 1962;88:86-90.

[33] Malamet M. Maximal hemostasis in suprapubic prostatectomy. *Surg. Gynecol. Obstet.* 1965;120:1307-1312.

[34] Cohen SP. Kopilnick MD, Robbins MA. Removable purse-string suture of the vesical neck during suprapubic prostatectomy. *J. Urol.* 1969;102:720-22.

[35] Nicoll GA, Riffle GN 2d, Andersen FO. Suprapubic prostatectomy. The removable purse string: a continuing comparative analysis of 300 consecutive cases. *J. Urol.* 1978;120:702-704.

[36] Denis R. Prostatectomy under depression. *J. Urol. Nephrol.* (Paris) 1970;76:663-72.

[37] Misop Han, Alan W. Partin: Retrograde and suprapubic open prostatectomy. In: Wein AJ, Kavoussi LR, Novick AC, Partin AW, Peters CA, editors. Campbell – Walsh Urology, ed. 9, Philadelphia, *Saunders Elsevier*, 2007. pp. 2845-2853.

[38] Ray E. Stutzman. In James F. Glenn, editor. *Urologic Surgery*, ed. 4, J.B. Lippincott, Philadelphia, 1991. pp 585-602.

[39] Flocks RH: The arterial distribution within the prostate gland: its role in transurethral prostatic resection, *J. Urol.* 1937;37:524.

[40] Clegg EJ. The vascular arrangements within the human prostate gland. *BJU* 1956;28:428-35.

[41] Bilhim T, Pisco JM, Furtado A, et al. Prostatic arterial supply: demonstration by multirow detector angio CT and catheter angiography. *Eur. Radiol.* 2011;21:1119-1126.

[42] Takeuchi M, Masumori N, Tsukamoto T. Contemporary patients with LUTS/BPH requiring prostatectomy have long-term history of treatment with alpha 1-blockers and large prostates compared with past cases. *Urology* 2009; 74(3): 606-9.

In: Prostatectomies
Editors: H. Alvelos and Y. Izidoro
ISBN: 978-1- 62081-077-4
© 2012 Nova Science Publishers, Inc.

Chapter III

Diagnosis and Management of Post Prostatectomy Incontinence

***Etai Goldenberg*[1], *Lawrence L. Yeung*[2] *and H. Henry Lai*[1,3*]**

[1]Division of Urologic Surgery, Department of Surgery, Washington University School of Medicine, St Louis, US
[2]Department of Urology, University of Florida, Gainesville, US
[3]Department of Surgery, St Louis Veterans Affairs Medical Center, St Louis, US

Abstract

Urinary incontinence can occur after surgery for benign and malignant diseases of the prostate, including radical prostatectomy and endoscopic prostate surgery. Most often the incontinence is mild or transient, however if it is severe or persists, the incontinence can have detrimental effects on patient's quality of life. Thorough evaluation of the patient with a detailed history, physical examination, and diagnostic studies is necessary to formulate the diagnosis and tailor the treatment.

[*] Corresponding Author: H. Henry Lai, MD. Division of Urologic Surgery, Department of Surgery, Washington University School of Medicine, St Louis MO 63110, US.

The focus of this chapter is on the evaluation and treatment of post-prostatectomy stress urinary incontinence.

Epidemiology

The reported incidence of incontinence after prostatectomy ranges from 5% to 87% in the literature. The rate varies depending on the definition used to define incontinence, the method used to obtain and quantify the data, timing after surgery, patient selection, the stage of prostate cancer, surgical approach or technique, and adjuvant treatment.

The definition of continence varies among studies, from total urinary control, to social continence (wearing one or less safety pads per day). Patients report higher rates of incontinence on written questionnaires than face-to-face evaluation with a provider.

Additionally, patients report higher rates of incontinence than physicians. [1-3] Between 20-30% of patients report some degree of permanent incontinence in contemporary studies. [4-6] Overall, it appears that incontinence rates are lower with nerve-sparing radical prostatectomy with rates of 6-19%. There has not been a demonstrated difference in continence rates between open, laparoscopic, or robotic surgical approaches. [1, 2]

Younger patients have faster and more complete return of continence after surgery. The rates of incontinence increase with the age of the patient at the time of surgery.

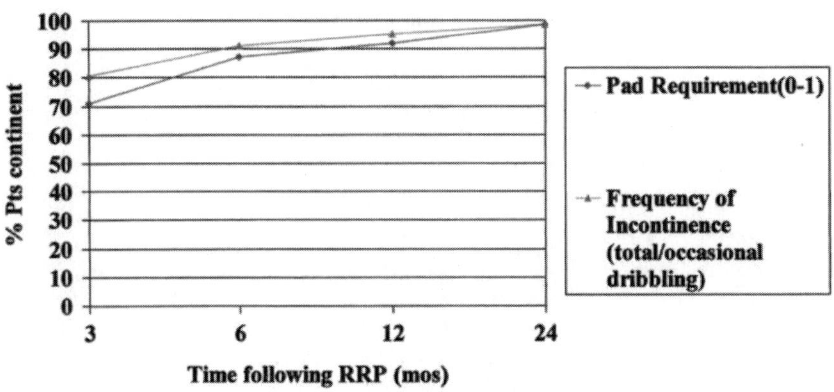

Figure 1. Incontinence rate decreases with time after radical prostatectomy. [8].

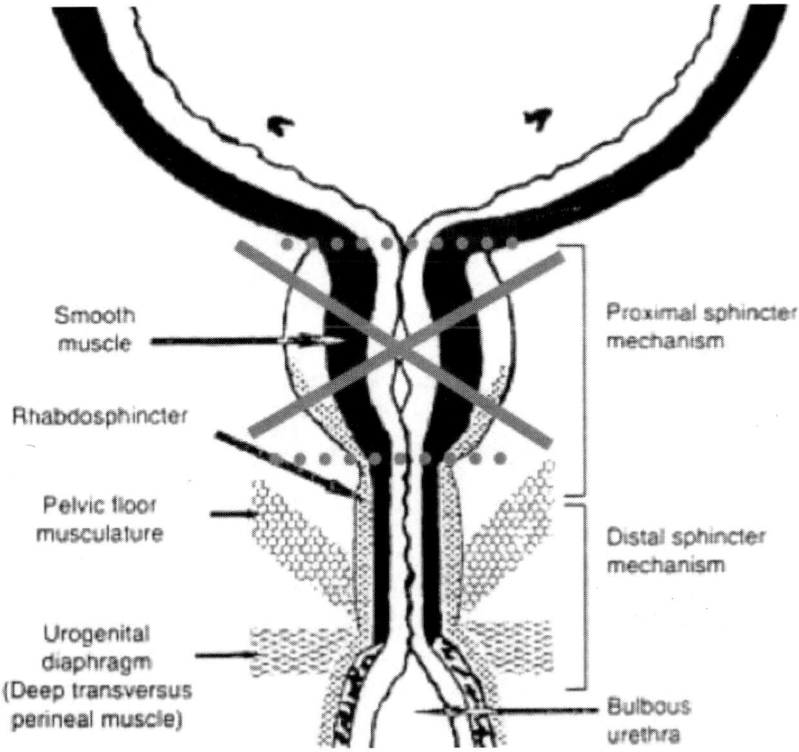

Figure 2. Anatomy of the internal (proximal) and external (distal) urinary sphincters. Stress incontinence results when both urinary sphincters are compromised after prostatectomy.

Each decade of life has a 2-fold increase in incontinence rates starting with surgery performed for a patient in his 50's. [7, 8] Patients who are overweight or who have preoperative impotence have also been found to have decreased continence rates. [9]

The return of continence after prostatectomy is time dependent. Following prostatectomy, all patients initially have some degree of incontinence. Lepor *et al.* found that by six months, around 87% of patients had achieved continence; however the rate continued to improve up to two years after the surgery, with 92% continence at 12 months and 98% at 24 months (Figure 1). [2, 3, 8]

Salvage radiation therapy is another risk factor for urinary incontinence, with approximately half of patients reporting and 40% undergoing treatment for incontinence. [10]

Anatomy

The human urinary sphincter is comprised of two distinct components: the internal and external urinary sphincters (Figure 2). At least one of the two sphincters needs to be functional in order to maintain continence. The internal urinary sphincter is composed of smooth muscle and is located at the bladder neck and the most proximal portion of the urethra. The external urinary sphincter is composed of striated muscle and is located at the membranous portion of the urethra. During prostatectomy, the internal urinary sphincter is surgically removed, leaving only the external urinary sphincter to maintain continence. Post-prostatectomy incontinence can be caused by direct surgical trauma to the muscles of the sphincter, injury to the nerves supplying the sphincter, or by unmasking pre-existing deficits of the external sphincter. This loss leads to intrinsic sphincter deficiency (ISD) and post-prostatectomy stress incontinence.

Men may also have underlying bladder dysfunction or detrusor overactivity (DO, involuntary bladder contractions), which can contribute to post-prostatectomy urge incontinence. Often, both stress and urinary incontinence (called mixed incontinence) exist. However, ISD is most often the cause of post-prostatectomy incontinence. A review of urodynamic findings of men after prostatectomy showed that 90% of patients had ISD contributing to their incontinence. Bladder dysfunction was the sole cause of incontinence in only 3% of the patients and contributed to the symptoms in 27% (ISD plus DO). [11]

Diagnosis and Evaluation

A thorough history is vital to evaluating the patient with post-prostatectomy urinary incontinence. History should be taken to ascertain the description of incontinence/voiding patterns, alleviating and aggravating factors, how symptoms have evolved since surgery, and the degree of bother to the patient. Use of validated questionnaires is also recommended to assess a patient's incontinence/voiding pattern. [12] Further insight into the patient's symptoms can be obtained by having the patient record a 3-day voiding diary to document the frequency and triggers of leakage. A complete medical and surgical history should inquire specifically about the timing and type of prostate surgery, any previous or subsequent radiation therapy to the pelvis, and any neurologic conditions. All prescription, over the counter, and herbal medications should be reviewed to determine if any of these might be contributing to the continence.

Assessment should include a focused physical examination (general, genitourinary, and neurologic exam). Aspects of the general exam should focus on assessing mental status, dexterity, gait, cognition, and body habitus. The abdomen should be palpated to evaluate for any masses, a full bladder, and surgical scars. [12] Genitourinary examination should include a digital rectal examination to assess for disease recurrence, rectal tone (which signifies the integrity of the sacral nerves), and the bulbospongiosus reflex. This reflex is elicited by squeezing the glans penis and assessing if the perineum and anal sphincter contracts. Lack of reflex may be associated with a neurologic lesion. [13] Deficits on neurologic examination may suggest a neurogenic bladder.

A standing cough test should be performed to document the presence of stress incontinence, and determine the severity of the incontinence (e.g. gravity dependent continuous leakage). The patient stands upright with the feet shoulder width apart and is asked to cough or perform the Valsalva maneuver with a half-full bladder. A pad test may also be used to record the wet weight of incontinence pads over a 24-hour period to quantify the severity of incontinence.

A urinalysis should be routinely performed to screen for urinary tract infection. Uroflowmetry, which assesses the maximal flow rate (Q_{max}), may screen for bladder outlet obstruction (e.g. due to bladder neck contractures) or valsalva voiding (hypocontractile bladder). Overflow incontinence and urinary retention can be ruled out with bladder ultrasound or urethral catheterization.

Patients contemplating artificial urinary sphincter (AUS) or male sling surgery must undergo office cystoscopy to rule out bladder neck contracture or urethral stricture. Up to 36% of open radical prostatectomy patients with significant post-prostatectomy incontinence who planned for AUS placement were found to have a bladder neck contracture during preoperative cystoscopic evaluation. [14] The contracture/stricture must be addressed prior to AUS or male sling surgery. A contracture or stricture that has been incised must also remain patent for at least 3 months prior to AUS/sling implant, since about 25% of patients had recurrence within 3 months after the initial incision. [14] Patients contemplating transobturator (AdVance) sling surgery should also undergo cystoscopy to confirm that the membranous urethra is mobile, non-scarred, and residual sphincteric function is present (i.e. the sphincter coapts well and demonstrates concentric voluntary contraction with a duration for at least a few seconds). [15] Failure to demonstrate residual sphincteric function predicts AdVance sling failure. [16]

Urodynamics is a test where the bladder is filled through a pressure-sensing catheter and pelvic floor activity is monitored through electromyography. This test can be used to evaluate bladder capacity, contractility, compliance, sensation, overactivity, urethral competence, and the pressure/flow relationship. Urodynamics is used to determine the etiology of the incontinence, to differentiate leakage of urine due to bladder dysfunction, ISD, or both, and to identify features that would adversely impact the outcome of surgical treatment (e.g. implanting an artificial urinary sphincter in patients with poor detrusor compliance and high storage pressure will put the upper tracts at risk after surgery). This information is useful to counsel patient expectation, and tailor treatment options.

Conservative Treatment of Urinary Incontinence

After prostatectomy, conservative therapies are initially used to manage the incontinence. Since the majority of patients achieve continence over time, leakage is initially managed by diapers, pads, or penile clamps. As the incontinence improves, these measures may be discontinued. If incontinence persists beyond 6 to 12 months, the numbers of protective pad use and the degree of bother to the patient are assessed to determine future interventions.

Behavioral therapies have become the mainstay empirical treatment for post-prostatectomy incontinence in the early postoperative period. Pelvic floor muscle exercises were first described by Kegel to improve stress incontinence in women. [17] Kegel exercises or Pelvic Floor Musculature Therapy (PFMT) appears to be beneficial in the initial management of post-prostatectomy incontinence. Patients randomized to receive formal PFMT have earlier return of continence compared to patients randomized to no PFMT instruction. Improved continence was seen at one and six months; however by one year after surgery, the rates were similar, leading to the conclusion that the PFMT only facilitates a faster time to recovery. [18, 19] Electro-stimulation with PFMT has not been found to improve incontinence. [20] Other behavioral modifications may also impact continence are timed voiding, and voiding prior to activities that may exacerbate incontinence.

Bladder dysfunction contributes to postoperative incontinence in about a quarter of patients. The patient's symptoms, physical exam or urodynamic findings will be compatible with urge incontinence and detrusor overactivity. Treatment of urge incontinence is achieved with behavioral modifications (timed voiding, PFMT, and avoidance of bladder irritants, such as caffeine, soda, citrus, citrus juices, spicy food, and artificial sweeteners). Anticholinergic medications may be given to manage urge incontinence if there is no obstruction.

Surgical Treatments for Post-prostatectomy Incontinence

Men who suffer from stress incontinence after prostatectomy may be candidates for anti-incontinence procedures such as bulking agent injection, male sling placement or artificial urinary sphincter (AUS) placement. For the male patient with significant stress incontinence, the artificial urinary sphincter is considered the gold standard surgical treatment because of the well-established success rates, outstanding patient satisfaction, long term durability, and acceptable complication rates demonstrated consistently in multiple longitudinal series with large numbers of patients. [14, 21-30] However, patients with milder degree of stress incontinence may opt for less invasive options. Surgical intervention of any type should be delayed for at least six months, optimally one year, after prostate surgery to allow for recovery of sphincteric function.

Peri-Urethral Bulking Agents

Men with mild stress incontinence who want to achieve social continence with minimally invasive (office based) procedures may consider peri-urethral injection. Injection of material into the submucosa near the bladder neck allows the tissue to coapt, increasing outlet resistance, and is done via an endoscopic/transurethral approach (Figure 3). Glutaraldehyde cross-linked collagen (Contigen) has been FDA-approved for the treatment of stress incontinence due to ISD since 1993. Unfortunately, the results are suboptimal and not durable.

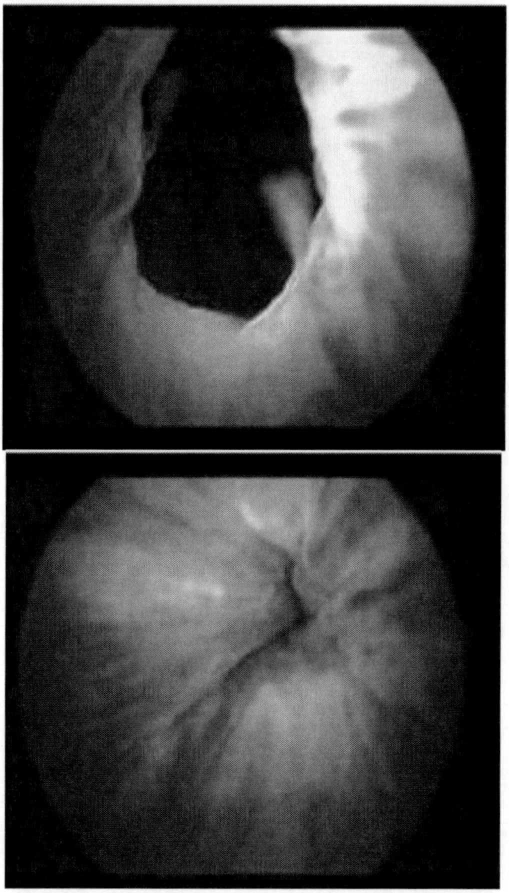

Figure 3. Peri-urethral bulking agent (before and after injection).

Smith *et al.* reported on a series of 62 men with post-prostatectomy incontinence that were treated with a peri-urethral collagen bulking agent. Only 8.1% of patients were totally dry, and 38.7% were socially continent (≤ 1 pad per day), while needing a median of 4 injection procedures to achieve social continence. [31] Westney *et al.* reviewed their results in 322 men and showed that incontinence improved from an average of five pads per day before injection, to only three pads per day after injection. [32] Only 17% achieved complete continence.

Additionally, the collagen was only durable for a mean of 6.3 months. Calcium hydroxylapatite (Coaptite), a newer peri-urethral bulking agent, provides more durable results than collagen in a randomized study that compared the efficacy of collagen and coaptite. [33] Silicone microimplant (Macroplastique) also appears to be better than collagen in a randomized trial. [34] Carbon-coated zirconium beads (Durasphere) have not shown any benefit over collagen. [35] Despite these studies, peri-urethral bulking agents are generally considered to have lower cure rates and suboptimal long-term success compared to the AUS or male slings. [36] It may have a role in patients with very mild stress incontinence or who is too ill to undergo surgery under anesthesia.

Male Slings

Kaufman described the use of surgical procedures to apply compression to the urethra to treat post-prostatectomy incontinence in the early 1970s. The crural bodies were crossed over or sutured together to apply compression to the bulbar urethra to prevent urinary leakage. [37] However, these techniques fell out of favor because of low success rates and high complication rates.

The sling concept was revived with the development of male bulbourethral slings made of polypropylene monofilament mesh that can be placed in a less invasive fashion. The exact mechanism of action of male perineal slings is unclear. It is thought that these slings place the bulbar urethra back in the normal anatomical position after radical prostatectomy, increase the functional length of the urethra, and limit movement of the urethra during valsalva, which diminishes incontinence. In contrast to the artificial urinary sphincter, which provides circumferential compression of the urethra, these slings provides one-directional vector compression on the urethra at all times. The two devices in the US with the most data available (albeit limited because of the newness of the devices) are the AdVance (transobturator) and InVance (bone-anchored perineal) sling systems (American Medical Systems, Minnetonka, MN, USA).

The InVance sling (Figure 4) is a bone-anchored polypropylene sling that is attached to the descending pubic rami with titanium screws and stretches across the bulbar urethra to compress it. Overall, 55-65% of patients reported complete dryness, and 23% decreased their pad usage by half after surgery. [38-40] Intermediate-term results (minimal 24 months follow-up) were acceptable. [40] However, 32% of men had no change in incontinence or were worse, and 73% had significant short-term perineal pain that resolved typically in 2 to 3 months.

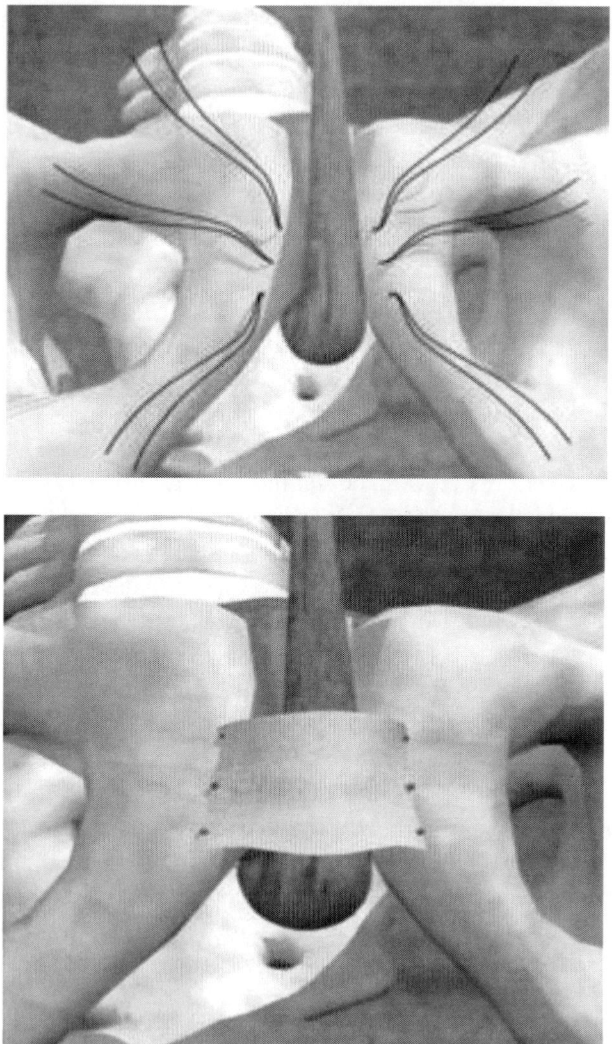

Figure 4. InVance bone-anchored male sling.(American Medical Systems, Minnetonka, MN, US).

For patients who failed inVance sling surgery, the artificial urinary sphincter may be safely implanted as a salvage procedure with good success. [41]. The AdVance sling (Figure 5) consists of two polypropylene mesh arms that are placed across the bulbar urethra via a transobturator approach using specially designed helical trocars.

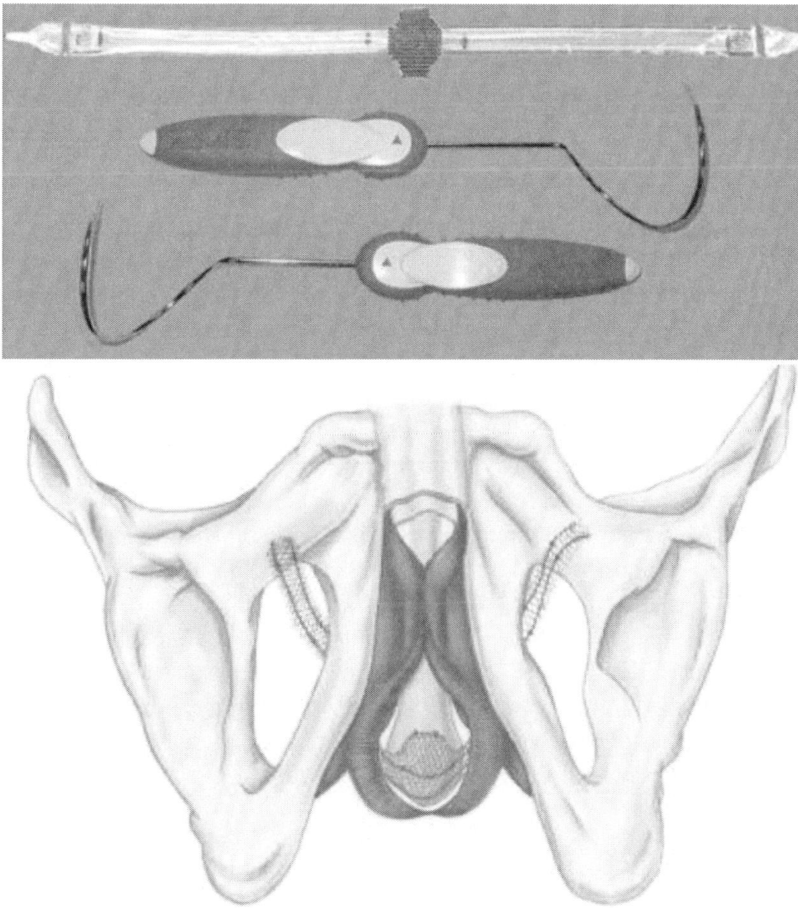

Figure 5. AdVvance transobturator male sling.(American Medical Systems, Minnetonka, MN, US).

Patients contemplating transobturator sling surgery should undergo office cystoscopy preoperatively to confirm that the membranous urethra is mobile, non-scarred, and residual sphincteric function is present (i.e. the sphincter coapts well and demonstrates concentric voluntary contraction with a duration for at least a few seconds). [15] Poor residual sphincter function and incomplete closure of the sphincter preoperatively are independent risk factors of surgical failure. [16] Early results showed complete continence rates ranging between 9-74% and an improvement of continence ranging between 17-45%. [15, 42-47] However, the results can be quite unpredictable and variable, with about 20-40% of men reporting either no change or worsened incontinence after surgery. Unlike the InVance sling, postoperative perineal pain is rare with the AdVance sling. Sling complication such as transient urinary retention (~20%) has been reported. [48] Mesh erosion into the male urethra appears to be uncommon. [49]

Intermediate-term results are beginning to emerge in the literature (minimum 20 months follow-up), and the results are quite acceptable overall (52% “cured”, 24% “improved”). [46] Patients who developed recurrent stress incontinence after AUS surgery (e.g. from urethral atrophy) may be salvaged with transobturator sling placement instead of cuff revision. [50] Patients who failed an transobturator sling may be managed with AUS or a repeat AdVance sling. [51]

The minimally invasive nature of the male sling is attractive to patients who are averse to the idea of having to operate an artificial sphincter. [52] Not having a mechanical device to manipulate or hydraulic components that may malfunction with time is another plus. However, proper patient selection is key in maximizing chances of success with male slings.

The ideal candidate for an AdVance sling is a patient who has mild to moderate stress incontinence (1-3 pads per day, or <200 gram/day) [53], has residual sphincter function as demonstrated on cystoscopy, [16] and who has not been irradiated in the pelvis. [53] Studies with long-termlonger follow up and larger number of patients are needed to determine the durability and true long-term effectiveness of these male sling procedures.

The Artificial Urinary Sphincter (AUS)

The artificial urinary sphincter (AUS) consists of a fluid-filled inflatable cuff that is implanted circumferentially around the urethra to coapt the lumen (Figure 6). The cuff essentially replaces the function of a damaged external sphincter to restore continence.

During urine storage, the cuff is kept inflated and the urethra is circumferentially compressed. Cuff inflation is maintained by pre-set pressure inside a hydraulic system maintained by a pressure-regulating balloon. When patient is ready to void, he squeezes on the pump, which then cycles the fluid away from the cuff to the pressure-regulating balloon. The cuff deflates, the urethral opens, and urination commences. After a delay of 3 to 5 minutes, the cuff inflates automatically to close off the urethra after voiding is completed.

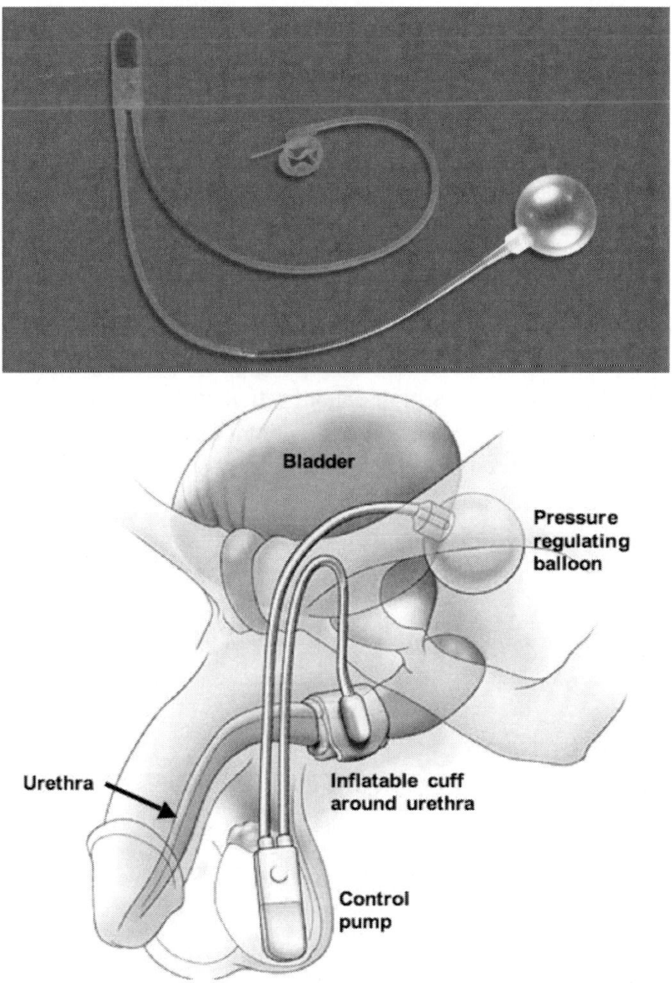

Figure 6. Placement of the artificial urinary sphincter (AUS). (American Medical Systems, Minnetonka, MN, US).

In 1972, F. Brantley Scott developed the first AUS that resembles the current model used today. The AMS 800 has undergone only minor revisions since the 1980s, including the use of a narrow-backed cuff to allow for more even distribution of fluid pressure around the urethra (1987), the use of kink-resistant and color-coded tubing for easier connection during surgery (1988), and antibiotics coating (minocycline plus rifampin) to reduce potential device infection and biofilm formation (2009).

The AMS 800 (American Medical System, Minnetonka, MN, USA) remains the lone artificial sphincter available in the US today. It can be customized to accommodate the urethra or bladder neck of men, women, and children with different cuff sizes (ranging from 3.5 cm to 11.0 cm) and pressure regulating balloons (41-50, 51-60, 61-70, 71-80, and 81-90 cm H_2Opressure).

The reported rate of complete urinary continence after AUS implantation varies between studies. However, "social continence", which is generally defined as requiring the use of no more than one incontinence pad per day, ranges from 59-90% after AUS placement (Table 1). [14, 21-30, 54] Patients with detrusor overactivity demonstrated on preoperative urodynamics or with overactive bladder symptoms (e.g. urgency) generally do well after AUS surgery. [55-60] The AUS has high patient satisfaction and improves patients' quality of life considerably. Over 90% of patients say that they would undergo the procedure again if needed. [61]

Table 1. Success rates of stress urinary incontinence treatment with the artificial urinary sphincter

Publication	No of patients	Mean follow-up (years)	Continence rates	Revision rates
Elliott *et al.* (1998)	313	5.7	Not reported	27%
Lai *et al.* (2007)	218	3.0	69%	27%
Montague *et al.* (1992)	166	3.5	75%	19%
Kim *et al.* (2008)	124	6.8	79%	29%
Venn *et al.* (2000)	100	11	84%	37%
Trigo Rocha *et al.* (2008)	40	4.5	90%	20%

The most common complications associated with AUS implantation are device infection, erosion, malfunction, and urethral atrophy (recurrent stress incontinence). The rate of device infection has been reported to be approximately 5.5% at a median of 3.7 months after surgery, the rate of erosion is about 6.0% at a median of 19.8 months after surgery, and the rate of device mechanical failure is 6.0% at a median of 68.1 months after surgery. [14] Urethral atrophy is the most common reason for stress incontinence to recur. These complications lead to the need for surgical revision of the device in 15-42% of patients (Table 1). [14, 24-30] Despite revisions, patients are satisfied with the AUS.

Conclusion

The reported rates of urinary continence after prostatectomy vary based on many factors such as the methods of reporting. Incontinence is most commonly caused by intrinsic sphincters deficiency. The appropriate evaluation requires a detailed history, physical exam, urinalysis, cystoscopy, and urodynamic studies. Postoperative stress incontinence usually improves with time and may be facilitated with pelvic floor rehabilitation.

When conservative measures fail after 6 to 12 months, patients should consider artificial urinary sphincter implantation (for moderate to severe stress incontinence), male sling procedures (for mild to moderate stress incontinence), or injectables (mild incontinence or non-surgical candidates). Although there are sparse long-term data on sling procedures compared to the AUS, male slings are appropriate for patients with less severe stress incontinence who understand the potential shortcomings of these procedures. The artificial urinary sphincter remains the gold standard treatment of more severe post-prostatectomy stress urinary incontinence.

Reference

[1] Evaluation and Management of Intrinsic Sphincter Deficiency after Radical Prostatectomy. *AUA Update*, 26, 2007.

[2] Eastham, J. A., Kattan, M. W., Rogers, E. et al.: Risk factors for urinary incontinence after radical prostatectomy. *J Urol,* 156: 1707, 1996.

[3] Lepor, H., Kaci, L., Xue, X.: Continence following radical retropubic prostatectomy using self-reporting instruments. *J Urol,* 171: 1212, 2004.

[4] Saranchuk, J. W., Kattan, M. W., Elkin, E. et al.: Achieving optimal outcomes after radical prostatectomy. *J Clin Oncol,* 23: 4146, 2005.

[5] Gaylis, F. D., Friedel, W. E., Armas, O. A.: Radical retropubic prostatectomy outcomes at a community hospital. *J Urol,* 159: 167, 1998.

[6] Hugosson, J., Stranne, J., Carlsson, S. V.: Radical retropubic prostatectomy: a review of outcomes and side-effects. *Acta Oncol,* 50 Suppl 1: 92, 2011.

[7] Catalona, W. J., Carvalhal, G. F., Mager, D. E. et al.: Potency, continence and complication rates in 1,870 consecutive radical retropubic prostatectomies. *J Urol,* 162: 433, 1999.

[8] Lepor, H., Kaci, L.: The impact of open radical retropubic prostatectomy on continence and lower urinary tract symptoms: a prospective assessment using validated self-administered outcome instruments. *J Urol,* 171: 1216, 2004.

[9] Loughlin, K. R., Prasad, M. M.: Post-prostatectomy urinary incontinence: a confluence of 3 factors. *J Urol,* 183: 871, 2010.

[10] Sanderson, K. M., Penson, D. F., Cai, J. et al.: Salvage radical prostatectomy: quality of life outcomes and long-term oncological control of radiorecurrent prostate cancer. *J Urol,* 176: 2025, 2006.

[11] Ficazzola, M. A., Nitti, V. W.: The etiology of post-radical prostatectomy incontinence and correlation of symptoms with urodynamic findings. *J Urol,* 160: 1317, 1998.

[12] Abrams, P., Andersson, K. E., Birder, L. et al.: Fourth International Consultation on Incontinence Recommendations of the International Scientific Committee: Evaluation and treatment of urinary incontinence, pelvic organ prolapse, and fecal incontinence. *Neurourol Urodyn,* 29: 213, 2010.

[13] Blaivas, J. G., Zayed, A. A., Labib, K. B.: The bulbocavernosus reflex in urology: a prospective study of 299 patients. *J Urol,* 126: 197, 1981.

[14] Lai, H. H., Hsu, E. I., Teh, B. S. et al.: 13 years of experience with artificial urinary sphincter implantation at Baylor College of Medicine. *J Urol,* 177: 1021, 2007.

[15] Rehder, P., Mitterberger, M. J., Pichler, R. et al.: The 1 year outcome of the transobturator retroluminal repositioning sling in the treatment of male stress urinary incontinence. *BJU Int,* 106: 1668, 2010.

[16] Soljanik, I., Gozzi, C., Becker, A. J. et al.: Risk factors of treatment failure after retrourethral transobturator male sling. World J Urol, 2011.

[17] Kegel, A. H.: Physiologic therapy for urinary stress incontinence. *J Am Med Assoc,* 146: 915, 1951.

[18] Filocamo, M. T., Li Marzi, V., Del Popolo, G. et al.: Effectiveness of early pelvic floor rehabilitation treatment for post-prostatectomy incontinence. *Eur Urol,* 48: 734, 2005.

[19] Parekh, A. R., Feng, M. I., Kirages, D. et al.: The role of pelvic floor exercises on post-prostatectomy incontinence. *J Urol,* 170: 130, 2003.

[20] Goode, P. S., Burgio, K. L., Johnson, T. M., 2nd et al.: Behavioral therapy with or without biofeedback and pelvic floor electrical stimulation for persistent postprostatectomy incontinence: a randomized controlled trial. *JAMA*, 305: 151, 2011.

[21] Gousse, A. E., Madjar, S., Lambert, M. M. et al.: Artificial urinary sphincter for post-radical prostatectomy urinary incontinence: long-term subjective results. *J Urol,* 166: 1755, 2001.

[22] Scott, F. B., Bradley, W. E., Timm, G. W.: Treatment of urinary incontinence by implantable prosthetic sphincter. *Urology,* 1: 252, 1973.

[23] Haab, F., Trockman, B. A., Zimmern, P. E. et al.: Quality of life and continence assessment of the artificial urinary sphincter in men with minimum 3.5 years of followup. *J Urol,* 158: 435, 1997.

[24] Venn, S. N., Greenwell, T. J., Mundy, A. R.: The long-term outcome of artificial urinary sphincters. *J Urol,* 164: 702, 2000.

[25] Trigo Rocha, F., Gomes, C. M., Mitre, A. I. et al.: A prospective study evaluating the efficacy of the artificial sphincter AMS 800 for the treatment of postradical prostatectomy urinary incontinence and the correlation between preoperative urodynamic and surgical outcomes. *Urology,* 71: 85, 2008.

[26] Montague, D. K.: The artificial urinary sphincter (AS 800): experience in 166 consecutive patients. *J Urol,* 147: 380, 1992.

[27] Kim, S. P., Sarmast, Z., Daignault, S. et al.: Long-term durability and functional outcomes among patients with artificial urinary sphincters: a 10-year retrospective review from the University of Michigan. *J Urol,* 179: 1912, 2008.

[28] Chung, E., Cartmill, R. A.: 25-year experience in the outcome of artificial urinary sphincter in the treatment of female urinary incontinence. *BJU Int,* 106: 1664, 2010.

[29] Vayleux, B., Rigaud, J., Luyckx, F. et al.: Female urinary incontinence and artificial urinary sphincter: study of efficacy and risk factors for failure and complications. *Eur Urol,* 59: 1048, 2011.

[30] Thomas, K., Venn, S. N., Mundy, A. R.: Outcome of the artificial urinary sphincter in female patients. *J Urol,* 167: 1720, 2002.

[31] Smith, D. N., Appell, R. A., Rackley, R. R. et al.: Collagen injection therapy for post-prostatectomy incontinence. *J Urol,* 160: 364, 1998.

[32] Westney, O. L., Bevan-Thomas, R., Palmer, J. L. et al.: Transurethral collagen injections for male intrinsic sphincter deficiency: the University of Texas-Houston experience. *J Urol,* 174: 994, 2005.

[33] Mayer, R. D., Dmochowski, R. R., Appell, R. A. et al.: Multicenter prospective randomized 52-week trial of calcium hydroxylapatite versus bovine dermal collagen for treatment of stress urinary incontinence. *Urology,* 69: 876, 2007.

[34] Ghoniem, G., Corcos, J., Comiter, C. et al.: Cross-linked polydimethylsiloxane injection for female stress urinary incontinence: results of a multicenter, randomized, controlled, single-blind study. *J Urol,* 181: 204, 2009.

[35] Lightner, D., Calvosa, C., Andersen, R. et al.: A new injectable bulking agent for treatment of stress urinary incontinence: results of a multicenter, randomized, controlled, double-blind study of Durasphere. *Urology,* 58: 12, 2001.

[36] Onur, R., Singla, A.: Comparison of bone-anchored male sling and collagen implant for the treatment of male incontinence. *Int J Urol,* 13: 1207, 2006.

[37] Kaufman, J. J.: Surgical treatment of post-prostatectomy incontinence: use of the penile crura to compress the bulbous urethra. *J Urol,* 107: 293, 1972.

[38] Guimarães, M., Oliveira, R., Pinto, R. et al.: Intermediate-term results, up to 4 years, of a bone-anchored male perineal sling for treating male stress urinary incontinence after prostate surgery. *BJU Int,* 103: 500, 2009.

[39] Giberti, C., Gallo, F., Schenone, M. et al.: The bone anchor suburethral synthetic sling for iatrogenic male incontinence: critical evaluation at a mean 3-year followup. *J Urol,* 181: 2204, 2009.

[40] Comiter, C. V.: The male perineal sling: intermediate-term results. *Neurourol Urodyn,* 24: 648, 2005.

[41] Fisher, M. B., Aggarwal, N., Vuruskan, H. et al.: Efficacy of artificial urinary sphincter implantation after failed bone-anchored male sling for postprostatectomy incontinence. *Urology,* 70: 942, 2007.

[42] Cornel, E. B., Elzevier, H. W., Putter, H.: Can advance transobturator sling suspension cure male urinary postoperative stress incontinence? *J Urol,* 183: 1459, 2010.

[43] Bauer, R. M., Mayer, M. E., Gratzke, C. et al.: Prospective evaluation of the functional sling suspension for male postprostatectomy stress urinary incontinence: results after 1 year. *Eur Urol,* 56: 928, 2009.
[44] Cornu, J. N., Sebe, P., Ciofu, C. et al.: The AdVance transobturator male sling for postprostatectomy incontinence: clinical results of a prospective evaluation after a minimum follow-up of 6 months. *Eur Urol,* 56: 923, 2009.
[45] Bauer, R. M., Soljanik, I., Fullhase, C. et al.: Results of the AdVance transobturator male sling after radical prostatectomy and adjuvant radiotherapy. *Urology,* 77: 474, 2011.
[46] Bauer, R. M., Soljanik, I., Fullhase, C. et al.: Mid-term results for the retroluminar transobturator sling suspension for stress urinary incontinence after prostatectomy. *BJU Int,* 108: 94, 2011.
[47] Cornel, E. B., Elzevier, H. W., Putter, H.: Can Advance Transobturator Sling Suspension Cure Male Urinary Postoperative Stress Incontinence? *The Journal of Urology,* 183: 1459, 2010.
[48] Bauer, R. M., Mayer, M. E., May, F. et al.: Complications of the AdVance transobturator male sling in the treatment of male stress urinary incontinence. *Urology,* 75: 1494, 2010.
[49] Harris, S. E., Guralnick, M. L., O'Connor, R. C.: Urethral erosion of transobturator male sling. *Urology,* 73: 443 e19, 2009.
[50] Christine, B., Knoll, L. D.: Treatment of recurrent urinary incontinence after artificial urinary sphincter placement using the AdVance male sling. *Urology,* 76: 1321, 2010.
[51] Soljanik, I., Becker, A. J., Stief, C. G. et al.: Repeat retrourethral transobturator sling in the management of recurrent postprostatectomy stress urinary incontinence after failed first male sling. *Eur Urol,* 58: 767, 2010.
[52] Kumar, A., Litt, E. R., K.N., B. et al.: Artificial urinary sphincter versus male sling for post-prostatectomy incontinence-what do patients choose? *J Urol,* 181: 1231, 2009.
[53] Cornu, J.-N., Sèbe, P., Ciofu, C. et al.: Mid-term evaluation of the transobturator male sling for post-prostatectomy incontinence: focus on prognostic factors. *BJU International,* 108: 236, 2011.
[54] Elliott, D. S., Barrett, D. M.: Mayo Clinic long-term analysis of the functional durability of the AMS 800 artificial urinary sphincter: a review of 323 cases. *J Urol,* 159: 1206, 1998.

[55] Ballert, K. N., Nitti, V. W.: Association between detrusor overactivity and postoperative outcomes in patients undergoing male bone anchored perineal sling. *J Urol,* 183: 641, 2010.

[56] Lai, H. H., Hsu, E. I., Boone, T. B.: Urodynamic testing in evaluation of postradical prostatectomy incontinence before artificial urinary sphincter implantation. *Urology,* 73: 1264, 2009.

[57] Perez, L. M., Webster, G. D.: Successful outcome of artificial urinary sphincters in men with post-prostatectomy urinary incontinence despite adverse implantation features. *J Urol,* 148: 1166, 1992.

[58] Thiel, D. D., Young, P. R., Broderick, G. A. et al.: Do clinical or urodynamic parameters predict artificial urinary sphincter outcome in post-radical prostatectomy incontinence? *Urology,* 69: 315, 2007.

[59] Trigo Rocha, F., Gomes, C. M., Mitre, A. I. et al.: A prospective study evaluating the efficacy of the artificial sphincter AMS 800 for the treatment of postradical prostatectomy urinary incontinence and the correlation between preoperative urodynamic and surgical outcomes. *Urology,* 71: 85, 2008.

[60] Lai, H. H., Boone, T. B.: Implantation of artificial urinary sphincter in patients with post-prostatectomy incontinence, and preoperative overactive bladder and mixed symptoms. *J Urol,* 185: 2254, 2011.

[61] Kahlon, B., Baverstock, R. J., Carlson, K. V.: Quality of life and patient satisfaction after artificial urinary sphincter. *Can Urol Assoc J,* 2011.

In: Prostatectomies
Editors: H. Alvelos and Y. Izidoro
ISBN: 978-1- 62081-077-4
© 2012 Nova Science Publishers, Inc.

Chapter IV

Minimally Invasive Radical Prostatectomy: International Perspective of Efficacy and Availability of New Technologies Compared to Open Conventional Approach

Marcos Tobias-Machado,
Felipe Brandão Corrêa de Araújo,
Eduardo S. Starling and Antonio C. L. Pompeo
Section of Urologic Oncology, Department of Urology, ABC Medical School, Santo André, São Paulo; Brazil

Abstract

Introduction: The surgical treatment of prostate cancer has evolved rapidly, driven by technological advances that have made minimally-invasive prostatectomy feasible. The contemporary surgical approaches are laparoscopic radical prostatectomy and robot-assisted laparoscopic radical prostatectomy that are considered standard modalities across

North America, Europe and other reference centers. Despite the widespread adoption of these new techniques there are few robust studies directly comparing the results of these techniques with the standard open radical prostatectomy. This review aim to discuss the current status of minimally- invasive prostatectomy focusing on peri-operative, oncological and functional outcomes, costs and availability in different centers worldwide.

Matherial and methods: Analysis of published literature in PUBMED and google academic utilizing laparoscopic radical prostatectomy and robotic radical prostatectomy as key words. Peri-operative data ,oncological control, continence and potency rates, costs and availability in several centers around the world were compared.

Results: Both pure laparoscopic and robotic surgery have a reduced blood loss and transfusion rate compared to open. Oncological and functional results seems to be similar to open considering several studies with less than 500 operated patients. Results emerging from larger series of experienced surgeons (more than 1000 operated cases) has showing that robotic surgery can promote less complications and better oncological and functional results than open approach. Robotic is more expensive than laparoscopic and open approachs. Robotic is the prefered technique in USA. In Europe, robotic and laparoscopic are having growing acceptance and in Asia and South America there are few robotic systems and centers utilizing minimally invasive approachs.

Conclusions: Minimally invasive approachs has potential to reduce surgical morbidity and improve operative, oncological and functional results as experience comes growing. Costs and availability of trained surgeons and robotic systems in some places are the limitations to worldwide dissemination of minimally invasive radical prostatectomy. Out of USA and Europe open radical prostatectomy is yet the prefered technique to treat localized prostate cancer.

Introduction

The first radical prostatectomy (RP) was performed by Young in 1905 becoming the first therapeutic modality used in the surgical treatment of prostate cancer. The RP is ideally suited for patients with localized cancer and a life expectancy of at least 10 years. There is no specific age limit for its realization, but many authors use to limit the age of 75 years. More recently, we have expanded the spectrum of indications to perform radical prostatectomy, also becoming one of the options in multimodal treatment of locally advanced disease because of its efficacy in the control of local complications of the disease.

The minimally invasive radical prostatectomy has demonstrated over the last decade great benefits for patients. The first laparoscopic radical prostatectomy (LRP) was performed by Schuessler et al in 1992 [1]. It was in 1999 that Guillonneau and Vallancien in Montsouris, France published an initial series of 65 patients with prostate cancer treated with LRP, this series showed the world that the procedure was feasible and reproducible [2].

In 2000, Binder and Kramer performed the first robot-assisted laparoscopic prostatectomy (RALP) in Germany [3]. Its introduction in the United States in the same year, Menon et al led to its progress and development leading to the dissemination and popularization [4]. Since then, RALP represents another alternative in the surgical treatment of prostate cancer.

The use of robot-assisted radical prostatectomy is growing every year. Between 2005 and 2006 there was an estimated increase of 100% reaching about 40% of radical prostatectomies performed in the U.S. In 2011 this rate was estimated at 80%. However, this is not the reality all around the world.
The costs with the robotic systems are to hi and several centers were the pure laparoscopic radical prostatectomy is commonly performed it becomes the minimally invasive alternative to open procedure.

In the other hand others continents like Asia, Africa and most of Latin American countries, the open radical prostatectomy is still the surgical treatment most used for the treatment of localized prostate cancer.

Despite the wide diffusion of these treatment modalities there are only few studies comparing perioperative, oncologic and functional outcomes on minimally invasive radical prostatectomy with open radical prostatectomy (ORP).

Material and Methods

To carry out this chapter, an extensive literature review from 2000 to 2011 was conducted in Medline, PubMed and Google Scholar using laparoscopic and robotic radical prostatectomy as key words. Perioperative data, oncologic control, continence and potency rates, costs and availability in several centers around the world were analysed.

Perioperative Data and Postoperative Morbidity

Operative Time

When evaluating results of operative time in centers with extensive experience (more than 350 surgeries), open surgery has an average time of 165 min (131-204min), laparoscopic surgery 205 min (100-266min) and robotic surgery 162 min (130-236 min) [5].

According to the only randomized control trial comparing LRP and ORP the operative time was longer in those patients undergoing LRP [6].

A systematic review of 37 comparative studies performed by Ficarra et al [7] showed that the average operating time of RALP and LRP is superior to open radical prostatectomy, but that such difference disappeared passed the earlier phase of the learning curve, especially when analysed larger robotic cohort in high-volume surgical centers [8-10].

Blood Loss and Transfusion Rates

Less bleeding and lower blood transfusion rates are considered advantages of laparoscopic radical prostatectomy (LRP) and RALP when compared to ORP. Since most of the intraoperative blood loss stems from venous sinuses, the tamponade effect created by the pneumoperitoneum clearly helps to reduce bleeding.

In randomized analysis comparing LRP and ORP Guazzoni et al showed lower rate of bleeding with laparoscopic surgery (257ml x 853 ml) [6]. In a paired analysis comparing 120 RALPs with 240 ORP, Rocco and cols recently confirmed that blood loss during RALP is significantly lower when compared with ORP (200 ml vs. 800ml) [13].

Two recent meta-analysis including studies that directly compared ORP, LRP, and RALP confirmed that RALP and LRP are associated with less blood loss and less risk of transfusion when compared to open radical prostatectomy [7,14]. Parsons et al demonstrated that when minimally invasive techniques are used, the chance of blood transfusion is 77% lower when compared with open surgery [14].

Complication Rate

Surgical complications were documented in several publications of radical prostatectomy, but few studies used standardized classification systems. The lack of consensus within the surgical community regarding the best method to report complications can prevent accurate comparisons between different series and techniques.

Lepor et al reported an overall incidence of complications of 6.5% in a series of 1000 ORPs performed by one surgeon [15]. But in this case study, blood transfusion (9.7%) was not considered a complication. Most of the recently published series of RALPs and LRPs considers blood transfusion within the overall rates of complication. Thus, any direct comparison becomes inaccurate.

Meta-analysis published by Ficarra et al demonstrated similar rate of complications between the LRP and ORP [7]. Regarding the comparison between ORP and RALPs, Krambeck et al recently demonstrated a comparable perioperative complication rate (8.0% vs. 4.8%) [10]. Similarly, Nelson et al demonstrated equivalent rates of unscheduled visits (10%) and hospitalizations (ORP = 5% vs RALP = 7%) due to postoperative complications between these two surgical approaches [16].

Hu et al compared intraoperative and early postoperative complications of successive 358 LRPs and 322 RALPs and showed lower overall rates of complications after RALP (27.7%vs. 14.6%) [17]. In contrast, Rozet et al in paired analysis of 133 extraperitoneal RALPs and 133 extraperitoneal LRP, showed higher overall complication rate after robotic-assisted laparoscopic prostatectomy (19.4% vs.9.1%) [18]. Comparing outcomes in high-volume centers Coelho et al demonstrated similar complication rates between the techniques, ORP 10.3%, LRP 10.9% and 10.3% RALP [5].

Length of Hospital Stay

The length of hospital stay in samples of radical prostatectomy performed in the U.S. is usually lower when compared to European case studies, where patients often remain hospitalized until removal of the Foley catheter [19-26]. However, the average length of stay is significantly lower in patients undergoing minimally invasive radical prostatectomy over ORP in most comparative studies currently available in the literature. In a prospective study comparing 612 ORP and 818 LRP Touijer et al showed lower length of stay in the group submitted to LRP (2.0 x 3.2 days) [27].These data are corroborated by the meta-analysis published by Ficarra et al in which patients undergoing LRP were discharged on average 2.4 days earlier than patients undergoing ORP [7].

When analyzed studies about robotic radical prostatectomy Krakemberg et al in a paired analysis comparing 294 RALPs and 588 ORP, demonstrated length of hospital stay significantly shorter in the group undergoing RALP (29.3% vs 19.4% of patients with length of stay less than 1 day) [10] .Similarly, Rocco et al demonstrated mean hospital stay shorter after RALP compared to ORP (3 vs 6 days) [13].

Oncologic Outcomes

The primary goal of prostate cancer surgery is to provide satisfactory oncologic outcomes. Biochemical progression and margin positivity are the commonly used indices to assess oncologic outcomes following radical prostatectomy. An increasing prostate-specific antigen (PSA) level is an early sign of biochemical progression and prostate cancer recurrence. The surgical margin status is one of the most important results to be evaluated in any surgical treatment for prostate cancer. For patients with tumors confined to the prostate the PSA progression-free survival after 10 years is 85%, but this value drops to 55% when surgical margin is positive.

In a study evaluating surgical margins in 1389 patients undergoing ORP, Swindle et al showed positive surgical margin (PSM) rate of 12.9%. When analyzed by stage, these values were 6.8% for patients with pathologic stage pT2 and 23% for patients stage pT3 [29].

Regarding the comparison of positive surgical margin rates between the different surgical approaches (ORP, LRP and RALP) the results are conflicting. A systematic review of thirteen comparative studies showed no significant difference in overall incidence of positive margins between then [14]. In subgroup analysis according to tumor stage, also did not find any significant difference between groups for pT2 or pT3 tumors.

In the study with the highest level of evidence (1b), Guazzoni et al demonstrated that the positive surgical margin rates in ORP e LRP were overllaping [6].

Previous studies have shown that surgeon experience and the learning curve can affect the oncologic results after robotic radical prostatectomy.

Atugo et al evaluated 140 consecutive patients who underwent RALP by the same surgical team. Patients were divided into three groups based on the period in which surgery was performed: group I-the first 33 cases, group II included 33 intermediate cases, and group III - the last 34 cases. The positive margin rates were 45.4%, 21.2% and 11.7% for groups I, II, and III, respectively. The difference between the groups was statistically significant ($p = 0.0053$), showing lower rates of PSM with increasing experience of surgeons [30]. Similarly, Patel et al, evaluating 500 consecutive RALPs performed by a single surgeon, showed a positive surgical margin rate of 13% in the first 100 patients and 8% in the last 100 patients in the series.

Schroek et al, compared 362 RALPs with 435 ORPs and showed no significant difference in the incidence of positive margins between the groups. Adjusting according to clinical and pathological stage the risk of biochemical recurrence was not significantly different between groups [23]. Similarly, Krambeck et al in a paired comparison showed no difference in the rate of PSM between RALP and ORP.

The free biochemical recurrence rate at 3 years was not significantly different between groups (92.4% vs. 92.2%) [10]. Contrary to these results, Smith et al analyzed the results of 1747 patients undergoing radical prostatectomy (RALP in 1238 and ORP in 509) and selected the last 200 consecutive patients in each group. The result showed lower incidence of positive margins after RALP. Similarly, in a cumulative analysis of six comparative studies, Ficarra et al, demonstrated that the RALP was followed by a lower risk of positive margins compared with the ORP considering patients with localized cancer (stage pT2) [7].

Functional Outcomes

Urinary Continence

Compilation of data on different series including urinary incontinence is extremely difficult due to variations in definition, methods of data collection and follow-up. Very few data on urinary incontinence have been published in studies comparing ORP, LRP and RALP, so that definitive conclusions can not be obtained.

The paper by Touijer et al, showed a statistically significant difference in favor of ORP; patients undergoing LRP had a 2-fold higher risk of being incontinent [27]. However a cumulative analysis by Ficarra et al. and Toher et al suggests that the continence rates after ORP or LRP are similar [7,33].

Some recent studies suggested that continence can be achieved more quickly after RALP compared to ORP. Tewari et al compared 100 RALPs with 200 ORPs and demonstrated shorter time to recovery of continence after RALP (median 160 vs. 44 days) [34]. Similarly, Rocco et al demonstrated in a paired analysis, significantly better continence rates after RALP when compared to ORP. The rates of continence after RALP and ORP at 3, 6 and 12 months were 70%, 93%, 97% and 63%, 83%,88%, respectively [13].

In contrast to these results, Krambeck et al, in a paired comparison between ORP and RALP, showed comparable rates of continence between the two groups with postoperative follow-up of 1 year (91.8% x 93.7%) [10]. Also, Parsons and Bennet, analyzing rates of urinary incontinence one year after surgery in four comparative studies, found no significant difference between LRP and ORP or RALP [14].

Several technical modifications have been proposed to promote early return of continence after radical prostatectomy. Rocco et al recently described a technique for reconstruction of the posterior rhabdosphincter [35]. To avoid caudal retraction of the urethrosphincteric complex, before completing the vesicourethral anastomosis the posterior semicircumference of the sphincter is joined to the residuum of Denonvilliers' fascia and fixed to the posterior bladder wall 1 to 2 cm cranial and dorsal to the new bladder neck. Vesicourethral anastomosis is subsequently performed with care taken not to involve the neurovascular bundles. These authors reported early recovery of urinary continence after LRP and RALP using this technique [35, 36].

Recently, Coughlin et al reported encouraging preliminary results incorporating the posterior reconstruction technique after RALP. These authors reported a continence rate of 58% one week after RALP defined by the absence of pad usage [37].

Tewari et al described a technique for reconstruction of anterior and posterior (total reconstruction) during RALP. 214 patients received no additional methods to provide support to the vesico-urethral junction and served as a control group. 314 patients received an anterior reconstruction only, to provide additional vesico-urethral anastomotic support and 182 patients received the total reconstructive procedure. The percentage of patients who had achieved continence in the control group were: 13%, 35%, 50%, 62% and 82% at the 1,6,12,24 and 52-week follow-up, respectively. The percentage of patients who had achieved continence in the anterior reconstruction group were 27%, 59%, 77%, 86% and 91% respectively. The total reconstruction group had continence rates of 38%, 83%, 91%, and 97% at 1, 6, 12, and 24 weeks, respectively. At all the follow-up intervals the continence rate was significantly less in the control group than in the anterior reconstruction group and the total reconstruction group ($P < 0.01$) [38].

Recently, Patel et al described the technique of periurethral suspension during RALP and demonstrated statistically higher rates of continence 3 months after surgery compared to controls (without suspension) (92.8% vs. 83%) [39].

Sexual Function

Sexual function is one of the most difficult outcomes to assess after radical prostatectomy. Other factors beyond the surgeon or surgical approach have a significant effect on recovery of potency, as age of patient, baseline potency, baseline sexual activity, the stability of any relationship, cardiovascular comorbidities, the use of medications and the technique of "nerve-sparing" (NS). In addition, the evaluation of postoperative potency is not standardized, including non-validated questionnaires.

Previous studies have evaluated the importance of the technique used during dissection of the neurovascular bundle (NVB) for the recovery of sexual function after surgery. Finley et al analyzing the use of cautery during the NVB preservation demonstrated that the adoption of a cautery-free technique promoted potency rates significantly higher after surgery [28].

Kaul et al introduced the concept of complete preservation of the prostatic fascia (Veil of Aphrodite) in order to provide maximal preservation of nerve fibers. Prior to this, NVB preservation was performed in an "intraprostatic fascia" fashion. In one of the first studies comparing the "classic" NVB preservation with the "complete" prostatic fascia (or Veil of Aphrodite) preservation, 97% of patients at 12 months in the Veil of Aphrodite preservation group had erections strong enough for sexual intercourse compared with 74% in the "classic" NVB preservation group [40].

It is difficult based on the current literature to determine if one approach is superior to the other for the preservation of the neurovascular bundles and sexual function.

To date there are no comparative studies that show inferior results in terms of potency for LRP compared to ORP. Roumeguere et al in a prospective study showed similar potency rates in one year follow up between ORP and LRP[41]. In two meta-analysis published in the literature, Ficarra et al and

Parsons and Bennett showed no differences in potency rates at 12 and 18 months between laparoscopic and open techniques [7,14]. In a single institutional study, Abbou et al. reported similar potency rates at 3, 6 and 12 months for patients undergoing LRP and ORP [42].

When compared erectile function recovery after RALP and ORP the results are controversial. Paired analysis conducted by Krambeck et al showed that the potency rate at 1 year follow-up were comparable after RALP (70.0%) and ORP (62.8%) [10].

Tewari et al demonstrated earlier sexual recovery after RALP when compared to ORP. Patients who underwent RALP showed earlier return of erections (50% in a mean follow up of 180 days versus 50% in a mean follow up of 440 days after ORP) as well as a faster return to sexual intercourse (50% in 340 days after RALP versus 50% in 700 days for ORP) [34].

Although there are no comparative studies confirming the superiority of robotic surgery, technical modifications during NS has demonstrated very high rates of recovery of sexual function. Menon et al has recently described the "superveil" modification, sparing nerves in the posterolateral aspect as well as in the anterior aspect of the prostate between the 11 and 1 o'clock positions. In a report on 154 consecutive patients in whom this tissue was preserved, reported a 96% intercourse rate and a 69% normal erection rate at 12 months after surgery [43].

In a review, trying to minimize the potential bias of the initial learning curve, Coelho et al evaluated only the largest series published with the three surgical approaches. In this paper, evaluating RALP, they reported that the weighted mean potency rate at 12 months follow up for patients who underwent unilateral and bilateral nerve sparing, were 59.9% and 93.5% respectively. These values were higher than those found when the open and pure laparoscopic techniques were used (43.1% and 60.6% for ORP and 31.1% and 54% for LRP) [5].

Cost / Economics Considerations

The cost and economic issue must be considered when comparing the different approaches with radical prostatectomy. The da Vinci Surgical System costs approximately $ 1.6 million with a maintenance fee of $ 120.000/year after the first year. The financial responsibilities for starting and maintaining a robotic practice can be intimidating.

Lotan et al reported that ORP had a cost advantage of $487 over LRP and $1726 over RALP. According to the authors LRP has proved to be almost as cost competitive as ORP, whereas RALP is the most expensive to the hospital due to purchase of the robot, maintenance, and cost of operative equipment [44]. These finds were also demonstrated by Bolens et al [45]. On the other hand, Scales et al noted that the costs of robotic surgery depend on the number of surgeries performed. This study demonstrated that RALP could achieve cost equivalence with ORP at a surgical volume of 10 cases weekly. If case volume increased to 14 cases weekly, RALP would be less expensive than ORP [46]. Hohwu et al. suggested that a way to improve the cost effectiveness may be to perform RALP at fewer high volume urology centers and utilize the full potential of each robo [47].

Despite the costs are not apparently a problem in the U.S and some European countries, this is not reality of developing countries and the robotic surgery is a reality attainable by a small number of citizens and distant from the daily practice of the vast majority of urologists in these centers. Of more the 1800 robotic platforms worldwide, there are only 50 located in Asia, 15 in Latin America and none in Africa [48-50]. In this scenario the laparoscopic radical prostatectomy appears to be the minimally invasive option to open surgery when the robotic system is not available [51-53]. Maybe with time, reductions in costs will allow robotic technology to become a more established practice and achieve wider global acceptance and application.

Conclusion

Minimally invasive radical prostatectomy has potential to reduce surgical morbidity and improve operative, oncologic and functional results as experience comes growing. Costs and availability of trained surgeons and robotic systems in some places are limitations to worldwide dissemination of minimally invasive approach. Out of USA and Europe, open radical prostatectomy is yet the preferred technique to treat localized prostate cancer.

References

[1] Schuessler WWK, L.R.; Clayman, R.U. et al.. Laparoscopic Radical prostatectomy: initial case report. 1992. Located at: *J. Urol.*

[2] Guillonneau B, Vallancien G. Laparoscopic radical prostatectomy: initial experience and preliminary assessment after 65 operations. *Prostate.* Apr 1 1999;39(1):71-75.

[3] Binder J, Kramer W. Robotically-assisted laparoscopic radical prostatectomy. *BJU Int.* Mar 2001;87(4):408-410.

[4] Pasticier G, Rietbergen JB, Guillonneau B, Fromont G, Menon M, Vallancien G. Robotically assisted laparoscopic radical prostatectomy: feasibility study in men. *Eur Urol.* Jul 2001;40(1): 70-74.

[5] Coelho RF, Rocco B, Patel MB, Orvieto MA, Chauhan S, Ficarra V, Melegari S, Palmer KJ, Patel VR Retropubic, laparoscopic, and robot-assisted radical prostatectomy: a critical review of outcomes reported by high-volume centers.*J Endourol.* 2010 Dec;24(12): 2003-15.

[6] Guazzoni G, Cestari A, Naspro R, et al. Intra- and peri-operative outcomes comparing radical retropubic and laparoscopic radical prostatectomy: results from a prospective, randomised, single-surgeon study. *Eur Urol.* Jul 2006;50(1):98-104.

[7] Ficarra V, Novara G, Artibani W, et al. Retropubic, laparoscopic, and robot-assisted radical prostatectomy: a systematic review and cumulative analysis of comparative studies. *Eur Urol.* May 2009;55(5):1037-1063.

[8] Badani KK, Kaul S, Menon M. Evolution of robotic radical prostatectomy: assessment after 2766 procedures. *Cancer.* Nov 1 2007;110(9):1951-1958.

[9] Patel VR, Palmer KJ, Coughlin G, Samavedi S. Robot-assisted laparoscopic radical prostatectomy: perioperative outcomes of 1500 cases. *J Endourol.* Oct 2008;22(10):2299-2305.

[10] Krambeck AE, DiMarco DS, Rangel LJ, et al. Radical prostatectomy for prostatic adenocarcinoma: a matched comparison of open retropubic and robot-assisted techniques. *BJU Int.* Feb. 2009;103(4):448-453.

[11] Guillonneau B, Vallancien G. Laparoscopic radical prostatectomy: the Montsouris experience. *J Urol.* Feb 2000;163(2):418-422.

[12] Eden CG, Cahill D, Vass JA, Adams TH, Dauleh MI. Laparoscopic radical prostatectomy: the initial UK series. *BJU Int.* Dec 2002;90(9):876-882.

[13] Rocco B, Matei DV, Melegari S, et al. Robotic vs open prostatectomy in a laparoscopically naive centre: a matched-pair analysis. *BJU Int.* Oct 2009;104(7):991-995.

[14] Parsons JK, Bennett JL. Outcomes of retropubic, laparoscopic, and robotic-assisted prostatectomy. *Urology.* Aug 2008;72(2):412-416.

[15] Lepor H, Nieder AM, Ferrandino MN. Intraoperative and postoperative complications of radical retropubic prostatectomy in a consecutive series of 1,000 cases. *J Urol.* Nov 2001;166(5): 1729-1733.

[16] Nelson B, Kaufman M, Broughton G, et al. Comparison of length of hospital stay between radical retropubic prostatectomy and robotic assisted laparoscopic prostatectomy. *J Urol.* Mar 2007;177(3): 929-931.

[17] Hu JC, Nelson RA, Wilson TG, et al. Perioperative complications of laparoscopic and robotic assisted laparoscopic radical prostatectomy. *J Urol.* Feb 2006;175(2):541-546; discussion 546.

[18] Rozet F, Jaffe J, Braud G, et al. A direct comparison of robotic assisted versus pure laparoscopic radical prostatectomy: a single institution experience. *J Urol.* Aug 2007;178(2):478-482.

[19] Borin JF, Skarecky DW, Narula N, Ahlering TE. Impact of urethral stump length on continence and positive surgical margins in robot-assisted laparoscopic prostatectomy. *Urology.* Jul 2007;70(1): 173-177.

[20] Chan RC, Barocas DA, Chang SS, et al. Effect of a large prostate gland on open and robotically assisted laparoscopic radical prostatectomy. *BJU Int.* May 2008;101(9):1140-1144.

[21] Joseph JV, Rosenbaum R, Madeb R, Erturk E, Patel HR. Robotic extraperitoneal radical prostatectomy: an alternative approach. *J Urol.* Mar 2006;175(3 Pt 1):945-950; discussion 951.

[22] Mottrie A, Van Migem P, De Naeyer G, Schatteman P, Carpentier P, Fonteyne E. Robot-assisted laparoscopic radical prostatectomy: oncologic and functional results of 184 cases. *Eur Urol.* Sep. 2007;52(3):746-750.

[23] Schroeck FR, Sun L, Freedland SJ, et al. Comparison of prostate-specific antigen recurrence-free survival in a contemporary cohort of patients undergoing either radical retropubic or robot-assisted laparoscopic radical prostatectomy. *BJU Int.* Jul 2008;102(1):28-32.

[24] Wood DP SR, Dunn RL,et al. . Short-term health outcome differences between robotic and conventional radical prostatectomy2007:945-949. Located at: Urology.

[25] Zorn KC, Gofrit ON, Orvieto MA, et al. Da Vinci robot error and failure rates: single institution experience on a single three-arm robot unit of more than 700 consecutive robot-assisted laparoscopic radical prostatectomies. *J Endourol.* Nov 2007;21(11):1341-1344.

[26] Nelson B, Kaufman M, Broughton G, et al. Comparison of length of hospital stay between radical retropubic prostatectomy and robotic assisted laparoscopic prostatectomy. *J Urol.* Mar 2007;177(3): 929-931.

[27] Touijer K, Eastham JA, Secin FP, Romero Otero J, Serio A, Stasi J, Sanchez- Salas R, Vickers A, Reuter VE, Scardino PT, Guillonneau B Comprehensive prospective comparative analysis of outcomes between open and laparoscopic radical prostatectomy conducted in 2003 to 2005.*J Urol.* 2008 May;179(5):1811-7; discussion 1817.

[28] Finley DS, Rodriguez E, Jr., Skarecky DW, Ahlering TE. Quantitative and qualitative analysis of the recovery of potency after radical prostatectomy: effect of unilateral vs bilateral nerve sparing. *BJU Int.* Nov 2009;104(10):1484-1489.

[29] P. Swindle, J. A. Eastham, M. Ohori et al., "Do marginsmatter? The prognostic significance of positive surgicalmargins in radical prostatectomy specimens," *Journal ofUrology*, vol. 174, no. 3, pp. 903–907, 2005.

[30] Atug F, Castle EP, Srivastav SK, Burgess SV, Thomas R, Davis R. Positive surgical margins in robotic-assisted radical prostatectomy: impact *of learning* curve on oncologic outcomes. *Eur Urol.* May 2006;49(5):866-871; discussion 871-862.

[31] Patel VR, Thaly R, Shah K. Robotic radical prostatectomy: outcomes of 500 cases. *BJU Int.* May 2007;99(5):1109-1112.

[32] Smith JA, Jr., Chan RC, Chang SS, et al. A comparison of the incidence and location of positive surgical margins in robotic assisted laparoscopic radical prostatectomy and open retropubic radical prostatectomy. *J Urol.* Dec 2007;178(6):2385-2389; discussion 2389-2390.

[33] Tooher R, Swindle P, Woo H, Miller J, Maddern G Laparoscopic radical prostatectomy for localized prostate cancer: a systematic review of comparative studies. *J Urol* Jun 2006;175(6):2011-2017.

[34] Tewari A, Srivasatava A, Menon M. A prospective comparison of radical retropubic and robot-assisted prostatectomy: experience in one institution. *BJU Int.* Aug 2003;92(3):205-210.

[35] Rocco F, Carmignani L, Acquati P, et al. Restoration of posterior aspect of rhabdosphincter shortens continence time after radical retropubic prostatectomy. *J Urol.* Jun 2006;175(6):2201-2206.

[36] Rocco B, Gregori A, Stener S, et al. Posterior reconstruction of the rhabdosphincter allows a rapid recovery of continence after transperitoneal videolaparoscopic radical prostatectomy. *Eur Urol.* Apr 2007;51(4):996-1003.

[37] Coughlin G, Dangle PP, Patil NN, et al. Surgery Illustrated--focus on details. Modified posterior reconstruction of the rhabdosphincter:

application to robotic-assisted laparoscopic prostatectomy. *BJU Int.* Nov 2008;102(10):1482-1485.

[38] Tewari A, Jhaveri J, Rao S, Yadav R, Bartsch G, Te A, Ioffe E, Pineda M, Mudaliar S, Nguyen L, Libertino J, Vaughan D. Total reconstruction of the vesico-urethral junction.*BJU Int.* 2008 Apr;101(7):871-7.

[39] Patel VR, Coelho RF, Palmer KJ, Rocco B. Periurethral suspension stitch during robot-assisted laparoscopic radical prostatectomy: description of the technique and continence outcomes. *Eur Urol.* Sep 2009;56(3):472-478.

[40] Kaul S, Bhandari A, Hemal A, et al. Robotic radical prostatectomy with preservation of the prostatic fascia: a feasibility study. *Urology.* 2005;66(6):1261-1265.

[41] Roumeguere T, Bollens R, Vanden Bossche M, et al. Radical prostatectomy: a prospective comparison of oncological and functional results between open and laparoscopic approaches. World *J Urol.* May 2003;20(6):360-36.

[42] Anastasiadis AG, Salomon L, Katz R, Hosnek R, Chopin D, Abbou CC: Radical retropubic versus laparoscopic prostatectomy: a prospective comparison of functional outcome. *Urology*. 2003; 62:292-7.

[43] Menon M, Shrivastava A, Bhandari M, et al. Vattikuti Institute prostatectomy: technical modifications in 2009. *Eur Urol.* 2009;56(1):89-96.

[44] Lotan Y, Cadeddu JA, Gettman MT: The new economics of radical prostatectomy:cost comparison of open, laparoscopic and robotic assisted techniques. *J urol.* 2004; 172: 1431-5.

[45] Bolenz C, Gupta A, Hotze T, et al. Cost comparison of robotic, laparoscopic, and open radical prostatectomy for prostate cancer. *Eur Urol.* Mar 2010;57(3):453-458.

[46] Scales CD, Jr., Jones PJ, Eisenstein EL, Preminger GM, Albala DM. Local cost structures and the economics of robot assisted radical prostatectomy. *J Urol.* Dec 2005;174(6):2323-2329.

[47] Hohwü L, Borre M, Ehlers L, Venborg Pedersen K. A short-term cost-effectiveness study comparing robot-assisted laparoscopic and open retropubic radical prostatectomy.*J Med. Econ.* 2011;14(4):403-9. Epub 2011 May 23.

[48] Yip SKh, Sim HG. Robotic radical prostatectomy in east Asia: development, surgical results and challenges. *Curr Opin Urol.* 2010 Jan;20(1):80-5.

[49] Den Julio A, Ahlering TE, Korkes F, Lopes Neto CA, Tobias-Machado M, Pompeo ACLWroclawski ER. Robotic assisted radical prostatectomy: a different treatment for prostate cancer? *Einstein.* 2010; 8:381- 2.

[50] Colombo Jr JR,Andreoni C,Lemos GC,Fonseca Filho LL,Di Pietro DL,Pinto W,Sardenberg C,Campos AH,Teixeira JC,Camargo LFA,Cendoroglo Neto M. Robot-assisted radical prostatectomy in Brazil: preliminary results. *Einstein.* 2009; 7:488-9.

[51] Mariano MB, Tefilli MV, Fonseca GN, Goldraich IH: Laparoscopic radical prostatectomy: 10 years experience. *Int Braz J Urol.* 2009; 35: 565-71; discussion 571-2.

[52] Starling ES, Reis LO, Vaz Juliano R, Korkes F, Wanderlei Dos Santos M Jr, Lima Pompeo AC, Tobias-Machado M. Extraperitoneal endoscopic radical prostatectomy: How steep is the learning curve? Overheads on the personal evolution technique in 5-years experience. *Actas Urol Esp.* 2010. Jul; 34(7):598-602.

[53] Wattayang P, Nualyong C, Leewansangtong S, Srinualnad S, Taweemonkongsap T, Chaiyaprasithi B, Amornvesukit T, Phinthusophon K, Jitpraphai S, Thiptirapong B, Sujijantararat P, Soontrapa S. Laparoscopic radical prostatectomy: oncological and functional outcomes of 559 cases in Siriraj Hospital, Thailand *.J Med Assoc Thai*. 2011 Aug;94(8):941-6.

[54] Tobias-Machado M, Lasmar MT, Wroclawski ER.Retroperitoneoscopic surgery with extracorporeal uretero-ureteral anastomosis for treating retrocaval ureter. *Int Braz J Urol.* 2005 Mar-Apr;31(2):147-50.

[55] Tobias-Machado M, Forseto P Jr, Medina JA, Watanabe M, Juliano RV, Wroclawski ER.Laparoscopic radical prostatectomy by extraperitoneal access with duplication of the open technique. *Int Braz J Urol.* 2004 May-Jun;30(3):221-6.

In: Prostatectomies
Editors: H. Alvelos and Y. Izidoro
ISBN: 978-1- 62081-077-4
© 2012 Nova Science Publishers, Inc.

Chapter V

Biochemical Recurrence Following Radical Prostatectomy

***Manish I. Patel*[1] *and Nicholas A. Campbell*[2]**
[1]Urological Cancer Centre, University of Sydney
Westmead Hospital, Westmead, Australia
[2]University of Sydney, Westmead Hospital,
Westmead, Australia

Abstract

The risk of cancer recurrence after radical prostatectomy can be estimated using nomograms based on validated prognostic factors. Follow-up can then be tailored to a patient's risk. The diagnosis of recurrence after radical prostatectomy is made when the PSA is greater than 0.2ng/ml. After recurrence, the great dilemma is to determine whether the recurrence is localized or systemic. This can be determined by a variety of imaging modalities and examination of prostatectomy characteristics and PSA kinetics.

Management of a recurrence can be expectant or therapy with salvage radiotherapy or androgen ablation therapy depending on the likelihood of localized disease, patient health and expectations.

1. Diagnosis and Management of Cancer Recurrence after Radical Prostatectomy

Approximately 40% of men diagnosed with prostate cancer will undergo radical prostatectomy. Of these, 15% to 46% will manifest an asymptomatic PSA rise post-operatively suggesting recurrence of the cancer.

This chapter reviews the prognostication, definition, investigation and management of a recurrence of prostate cancer. Radical prostatectomy can be performed by the open retropubic approach, perineal approach, laparoscopic and robot assisted laparoscopic approach. Interestingly, the management of recurrence and rate of recurrence is the same irrespective of the type of radical prostatectomy performed.

1.1. Prognostication and Estimation of the Risk of recurrence Following Radical Prostatectomy

Following radical prostatectomy, the ability to predict a risk of recurrence for a particular patient is of vital importance as this will serve to counsel the patient, determine follow up regimes and well as potentially apply adjuvant therapy or entry into a clinical trial. The most common methods of predicting risk of recurrence is by placing the patient into a risk category based on a number of variables known to increase recurrence risk. An alternative method is the nomogram which will use algorithms incorporating multiple variables to calculate a probability of achieving a particular end-point such as biochemical recurrence. Both methods however use similar prognostic variables which increase risk of recurrence. These are outlined in Table 1.

Table 1. Prognostic variables associated with recurrence after radical prostatectomy

Factor
Gleason score in pathological specimen
Pathologic stage
Pre surgery PSA
Seminal vesical invasion
Lymph node invasion
Positive surgical margins

Table 2. Models for the prediction of biochemical recurrence after radical prostatectomy

Reference	Year	Prediction instrument	Prediction variables
Kattan et.al.[1]	1999	Nomogram	PSA, Gleason score, ECE, SM, SVI, LNI
Partin et.al [27]	1995	Risk catagorisation	PSA, Gleason score, ECE
D'Amico et.al.[28]	1998	Probability graph	PSA, Stage, Gleason score, SM
Blute et.al. [29]	2001	Risk catagorisation	Adjuvant therapy, Gleason score, PSA, SVI, SM
Moul [30]	2001	Risk catagorisation	PSA, race, stage, Gleason score
Freedland et.al. [31]	2004	Risk catagorisation	Gleason score, % positive cores, PSA

Extra capsular extension (ECE), Surgical Margin (SM), Seminal Vesical Involvement (SVI), Lymphnode invasion (LNI).

There are at least 16 models for predicting the likelihood of biochemical recurrence after radical prostatectomy. Some of the commonly used prediction tools are given in Table 2. The most widely used is the Kattan nomogram [1] which is available online (http://www.mskcc.org/mskcc/html/10088.cfm) or on PDA. This useful application will give a patient the likelihood of freedom from progression for 2,5,7 and 10 years.

1.2. Follow up Strategies Following Radical Prostatectomy

The percentage of men failing after radical prostatectomy varies with different series but overall is approximately 30%-40% at 5 years[2,3]. The risk of relapse after 5 years is reduced but still persistent, suggesting follow-up should be continued for a longer time. Follow up is important after radical prostatectomy because if cancer does recur than salvage therapies are available aimed at curative intent and early hormone therapy after biochemical failure can be started. In addition there are a number of non-cancer related complications for which it is also important to maintain follow-up.

Follow-up entails regular visits where a thorough history related to cancer recurrence and complications of radical prostatectomy should be taken. Physical examination also includes a rectal exam, as rarely a palpable tumour may be the first sign of recurrence. The follow-up should also include a PSA test. The measurement of PSA is the corner stone of follow-up after radical prostatectomy. PSA recurrence almost always precedes clinical recurrence, in many cases by many years, it is however still possible to get a recurrence without a PSA rise [4,5]. The schedule of follow-up has not been well studied and there is no consensus of the correct timings. A common schedule used by many urologists is 3 monthly visits for the first year, 6 monthly for the next 4 years and then yearly after that. Men at low risk for recurrence could have 6 monthly visits for the first year as well.

1.3. Making the Diagnosis of Cancer Recurrence after Radical Prostatectomy

1.3.1. Definition of Biochemical Recurrence

There has been considerable debate as to what level of PSA constitutes a true biochemical failure. Most urologists will use a cut-off value of greater then or equal to 0.2ng/ml on 2 consecutive occasions as outlined in the latest European Association of Urology [6,7]. At values below these cut-offs, detectable PSA has a reduced likelihood of continuing to rise (consistent with disease progression). For example, a post-operative PSA between 0.11 to 0.2ng/ml has only a 64% likelihood of rising further within a year [7]. The half-life of PSA in the serum is 3.15 days [8] so serum PSA should fall to undetectable levels by 30 days post surgery. The first PSA level should not be taken prior to this. If the first PSA determination post-operatively is greater than 0.4ng/ml, the presence of systemic disease is quite possible. In rare cases the PSA after prostatectomy will fail to reach undetectable levels, but remains stable at a level below 0.4ng/ml. It is quite possible that this PSA is not due to cancer recurrence but from retained benign prostate tissue [9]. Ultrasensitive PSA assays are capable of detection thresholds of 0.001 to 0.01ng/ml. They are not recommended for routine post-operative surveillance as they are yet of unproven value [6]. These assays may detect minute amounts of PSA originating from non-malignant prostatic sources [10] and generate problems with false positive results. It is also important to remember that recurrence can occur without a rise in PSA and usually represents aggressive disease.

1.3.2. Local Verses Systemic Disease

Once a PSA recurrence has been established, one of the most problematic aspects of evaluating patients is to determine whether the source of PSA is localised or from metastatic disease. The distinction is important because the presence of localised disease only, allows for salvage therapy directed at the prostatic fossa with intent to cure. In contrast, metastatic disease is treated palliatively with androgen ablation therapy initially. The incidence of isolated localised disease in men presenting with PSA recurrence after prostatectomy ranges from 4% to 53% [11-13].

A persistent PSA rise is thought be due to micrometastases or retained prostate tissue possibly secondarily to a positive surgical margin. Table 3 outlines various diagnostic modalities and their usefulness in distinguishing between local and systemic cancer recurrence. Digital rectal exam is very limited in its diagnostic utility. The prostatic fossa palpation is highly variable after radical prostatectomy and there is often postoperative scar making the diagnosis of local recurrence difficult. It should not be used alone to determine a management decision. Ultrasound guided biopsy of the prostatic fossa is not recommended routinely as there are substantial problems associated with it. Firstly, with the prostate absent, the site to biopsy is not known. The true sensitivity and the true false negative rate is also not known [6]. Additionally, if a local recurrence of prostate cancer is identified, it does not exclude the presence of concomitant systemic disease as well. Finally results of salvage radiation therapy to the prostatic fossa is equivalent whether the biopsies are positive or negative [14]. In asymptomatic men, the utility of computed tomography and bone scan has been poor for men with PSA recurrence after radical prostatectomy [15]. It has been recommended by some to use it when the PSA is greater than 10ng/ml or the PSA doubling time (PSADT) is less than 6 months but there is little evidence on this subject.

Table 3. Diagnostic modalities for distinguishing between local and systemic spread in patients with biochemical recurrence after radical prostatectomy

Diagnostic modality	Clinical Usefulness
Digital Rectal Exam	None
Ultrasound-guided biopsy	None
Computed tomography	Marginal, consider if PSA>10ng/ml or PSADT<6 months
MRI	Under investigation
Bone Scan	Marginal, consider if PSA>10ng/ml or PSADT<6 months
Radiolablelled PSMA antibody	Potentially useful. Further trials required.
Positron emission tomography	Under investigation. None to date.

Table 4. Pathological and PSA variables for distinguishing between local and systemic spread in patients with biochemical recurrence after radical prostatectomy

Variable	Local Recurrence	Systemic Recurrence
Gleason Score	≤6	>7
Lymph node invasion	No	Yes
PSA Doubling time	≥ 12 months	< 3-12 months
PSA velocity at 1 year	< 0.75ng/ml/yr	≥ 0.75ng/ml/yr
Seminal vesical invasion	No	Yes
Time to PSA recurrence after RRP	> 2 years	≤ 1 year

ProstaScint, is a monoclonal antibody to prostate specific membrane antigen (PSMA), which is radiolabelled.

PSA is increased in poorly differentiated and metastatic prostate cancer. Detection of metastatic disease using this imaging method has a sensitivity of approximately 62% [16]. Further larger studies are needed however to establish its true sensitivity and specificity. MRI and its role in prostate cancer is yet to be fully delineated but its use is ever increasing and is likely to be the imaging modality of choice for prostate cancer in the future[17]. Its ability to detect recurrence after a radical prostatectomy whether locally or distant is even less clear. To date there are mainly of case reports [18, 19] or systematic reviews of the literature [20] and at this stage remains experimental and should be used in selected cases. MRI with spectroscopy has also been compared to [(18)F] choline PET/CT in detecting local recurrence after biochemical recurrence[21]. This study indicated a potential benefit of MRI over PET scan for diagnosing local recurrence. Currently, the most common method of distinguishing local from systemic prostate cancer recurrence following radical prostatectomy, when PSA levels are still low, is to use a combination of various pathological and PSA variables. Table 4. outlines the variables associated with local and systemic recurrence.

1.3.3. Natural History of Biochemical Recurrence

The natural history of progression to boney metastasis and then to death after biochemical recurrence is highly variable but generally prolonged. In a study where 304 men with biochemical recurrence after radical prostatectomy, were followed for up to 15 years, only 34% developed bone metastases at a median of 8 years. These men with bone metastases were treated with androgen deprivation therapy and median time to death from prostate cancer was 5 years later [22].

The real challenge is to identify the men with biochemical recurrence who will progress rapidly and die early, so early treatment can be instituted. The Gleason score in the prostatectomy specimen and PSA kinetics have been useful for estimating time to developing metastases in men with biochemical recurrence. Table 5. shows the effect of Gleason score, time to PSA recurrence and PSADT on metastasis free survival at 3 and 5 years. Clearly a Gleason grade >7, PSA recurrence earlier than 2 years and a PSADT of <10 months portrays a poor prognosis. Once men have developed bone metastases, a large proportion will die of prostate cancer. Freedland et.al. have demonstrated that the PSADT is strongly predictive of death from prostate cancer [23]. This data shows that if the PSADT is >15months, no patients over a 15 year period died from prostate cancer.

Table 5. Estimation of metastasis free survival following biochemical recurrence after radical prostatectomy

			% metastasis free	
			3 year	5 years
All patients			78	63
Gleason score 5-7	Recurrence >2 years	PSADT>10m	95	86
		PSADT≤10m	82	69
	Recurrence ≤2 years	PSADT>10m	79	76
		PSADT≤10m	81	35
Gleason score 8-10	Recurrence >2 years	PSADT>10m	77	60
	Recurrence ≤2 years	PSADT≤10m	53	31

Adapted from Pound et.al.[22] and Laufer et.al.[11].

1.4. Treatment Options for Cancer Recurrence Following Radical Prostatectomy

Unfortunately, to date there is no prospective randomised data that showing that treatment of PSA recurrence, at any level or by any modality improves survival. Common treatments undertaken after a PSA recurrence include expectant management, salvage radiotherapy and androgen deprivation therapy. The treatment option chosen depends on the patient's likelihood of (1.) local verses systemic disease, (2.) cancer characteristics and rate of growth (PSA), (3.) patient's co-morbidities and life expectancy, (4.) side effects of treatment, (5.) patient's wishes.

1.4.1. Expectant Management

As there is no definitive evidence that treatment of a PSA recurrence (only) improves survival, and knowing that only half the men will develop a bone metastasis at 8 years or later [22], close monitoring is a very reasonable option for elderly men or those with multiple co-morbidities. If during this time men develop metastases, they can start androgen ablation therapy.

1.4.2. Salvage Radiotherapy

Salvage radiotherapy is treatment of the prostatic bed with the aim of curing a man who has a PSA recurrence. It should only be given to men who have a reasonable chance of having only localized disease based on tumour characteristics, PSA kinetics and imaging.

While there are no studies that show that salvage radiotherapy will improve survival, PSA response to salvage radiotherapy is generally about 50% [24]. There is however a large range of responses (12%-77%) depending on the post-prostatectomy pathology and PSA kinetics [24].

PSA responses are better if the Gleason score is less than 8 (less likelihood of systemic disease), the surgical margin status is positive (higher likelihood of a local source of PSA), the PSADT is long (less chance of metastatic disease) and the salvage radiotherapy is given at a low PSA, preferable <1.0ng/ml (low tumour burden) [24].

A man with a Gleason 6 prostate cancer with positive surgical margins, PSADT>10 months and starting salvage radiotherapy with a PSA < 2.0ng/ml has a 77% chance of PSA response. A man with a Gleason score of 8, starting salvage therapy with a PSA>2.0ng/ml has a 12% chance of PSA response. In summary, salvage radiotherapy is effective if given early to someone who has a high likelihood of localized recurrence.

Side effects of salvage radiotherapy are generally well tolerated. Approximately 20% of men previously continent will become mildly incontinent [25].

Approximately 50% of potent men will suffer declines in erectile function and a number of men may also develop urethral strictures or bladder neck contractures.

1.4.3. Androgen Deprivation Therapy

Androgen ablation therapy or "hormonal therapy" is often used to treat men with PSA recurrence or men who have established metastases from prostate cancer. Treatment by this method can either be by bilateral orchidectomy, LHRH agonists or antiandrogens such as cyproterone acetate or high dose bicalutamide. The treatments all have the final effect of reducing prostate cancer growth and inducing apoptosis by stopping testosterone induced prostate cancer growth. While this therapy is palliative only, as the PSA and cancer will eventually begin to grow there can be quite a long time period before death. Once men have developed bone metastases and then start androgen deprivation therapy, they will live on average 5 years[22]. Men with PSA recurrence only will live much longer than this on average.

There is controversy as to how early to institute androgen ablation therapy in men that have PSA recurrence and is the subject of a number of on-going clinical trials. Retrospective data does suggest that select men with aggressive disease who receive early androgen deprivation therapy for PSA recurrence do experience a delay in developing bone metastases [26]. There is no data however to show it improves survival.

1.5. Summary

PSA is a highly sensitive marker for the detection of recurrence after radical prostatectomy. When the PSA reaches $\geq$ 0.2ng/ml, a patient is considered to have a recurrence. The patient's prognosis and likelihood of localised verses systemic disease is highly dependent on the prostatectomy pathology as well as the time to PSA recurrence after prostatectomy and PSADT. If a patient is likely to have localised recurrence, he is eligible for salvage radiotherapy. If the patient has a high likelihood of systemic disease, androgen deprivation therapy or expectant management may be a more reasonable approach to treatment.

References

[1] Kattan MW, Wheeler TM and Scardino PT: Postoperative nomogram for disease recurrence after radical prostatectomy for prostate cancer. *J. Clin. Oncol.* 17: 1499-507, 1999.

[2] Walsh PC, Partin AW and Epstein JI: Cancer control and quality of life following anatomical radical retropubic prostatectomy: results at 10 years. *J. Urol.* 152: 1831-6, 1994.

[3] Kupelian P, Katcher J, Levin H, Zippe C and Klein E: Correlation of clinical and pathologic factors with rising prostate-specific antigen profiles after radical prostatectomy alone for clinically localized prostate cancer. *Urology.* 48: 249-60, 1996.

[4] Morgan WR, Zincke H, Rainwater LM, Myers RP and Klee GG: Prostate specific antigen values after radical retropubic prostatectomy for adenocarcinoma of the prostate: impact of adjuvant treatment (hormonal and radiation). *J. Urol.* 145: 319-23, 1991.

[5] Oefelein MG, Smith N, Carter M, Dalton D and Schaeffer A: The incidence of prostate cancer progression with undetectable serum prostate specific antigen in a series of 394 radical prostatectomies. *J. Urol.* 154: 2128-31, 1995.

[6] Swindle PW, Kattan MW and Scardino PT: Markers and meaning of primary treatment failure. *Urol. Clin. North Am.* 30: 377-401, 2003.

[7] Freedland SJ, Sutter ME, Dorey F and Aronson WJ: Defining the ideal cutpoint for determining PSA recurrence after radical prostatectomy. Prostate-specific antigen. *Urology.* 61: 365-9, 2003.

[8] Partin AW and Oesterling JE: The clinical usefulness of prostate specific antigen: update 1994. *J. Urol.* 152: 1358-68, 1994.

[9] Moul JW: Variables in predicting survival based on treating "PSA-only" relapse. *Urol. Oncol.* 21: 292-304, 2003.

[10] Diamandis EP and Yu H: Nonprostatic sources of prostate-specific antigen. *Urol. Clin. North Am.* 24: 275-82, 1997.

[11] Laufer M, Pound CR, Carducci MA and Eisenberger MA: Management of patients with rising prostate-specific antigen after radical prostatectomy. *Urology.* 55: 309-15, 2000.

[12] Han M, Partin AW, Pound CR, Epstein JI and Walsh PC: Long-term biochemical disease-free and cancer-specific survival following anatomic radical retropubic prostatectomy. The 15-year Johns Hopkins experience. *Urol. Clin. North Am.* 28: 555-65, 2001.

[13] Connolly JA, Shinohara K, Presti JC, Jr. and Carroll PR: Local recurrence after radical prostatectomy: characteristics in size, location, and relationship to prostate-specific antigen and surgical margins. *Urology.* 47: 225-31, 1996.

[14] Koppie TM, Grossfeld GD, Nudell DM, Weinberg VK and Carroll PR: Is anastomotic biopsy necessary before radiotherapy after radical prostatectomy? *J. Urol.* 166: 111-5, 2001.

[15] Okotie OT, Aronson WJ, Wieder JA, Liao Y, Dorey F, De KJ and Freedland SJ: Predictors of metastatic disease in men with biochemical failure following radical prostatectomy. *J. Urol.* 171: 2260-4, 2004.

[16] Quintana JC and Blend MJ: The dual-isotope ProstaScint imaging procedure: clinical experience and staging results in 145 patients. *Clin. Nucl. Med.* 25: 33-40, 2000.

[17] Sciarra A BJ, Bjartell A, Eastham J, Hricak H, Panebianco V, Witjes JA.: Advances in magnetic resonance imaging: how they are changing the management of prostate cancer. *Eur. Urol.*. 59: 962-77, 2011.

[18] Giannarini G ND, Thalmann GN, Thoeny HC.: Diffusion-Weighted Magnetic Resonance Imaging Detects Local Recurrence After Radical Prostatectomy: Initial Experience. *Eur. Urol.* , 2011.

[19] Bertagna F AM, Bosio G et al: Role of ^{11}C-choline positron emission tomography/computed tomography in evaluating patients affected by prostate cancer with suspected relapse due to prostate-specific antigen elevation. *Jpn. J. Radiol.* 6: 394-404, 2011.

[20] Martino P SV, Galosi AB, Consonni P, Trombetta C, Palazzo S, Maccagnano C, Liguori G, Valentino M, Battaglia M, Barozzi L.: Role of imaging and biopsy to assess local recurrence after definitive treatment for prostate carcinoma (surgery, radiotherapy, cryotherapy, HIFU). *World J. Urol.* 5: 595-605, 2011.

[21] Panebianco V SA, Lisi D, Galati F, Buonocore V, Catalano C, Gentile V, Laghi A, Passariello R.: Prostate cancer: 1HMRS-DCEMR at 3T versus [(18)F]choline PET/CT in the detection of local prostate cancer recurrence in men with biochemical progression after radical retropubic prostatectomy (RRP). *Eur. J. Radiol.*, 2011.

[22] Pound CR, Partin AW, Eisenberger MA, Chan DW, Pearson JD and Walsh PC: Natural history of progression after PSA elevation following radical prostatectomy. *Jama.* 281: 1591-7, 1999.

[23] Freedland SJ, Humphreys EB, Mangold LA, Eisenberger M, Dorey FJ, Walsh PC and Partin AW: Risk of prostate cancer-specific mortality following biochemical recurrence after radical prostatectomy. *JAMA.* 294: 433-9, 2005.

[24] Stephenson AJ, Shariat SF, Zelefsky MJ, Kattan MW, Butler EB, Teh BS, Klein EA, Kupelian PA, Roehrborn CG, Pistenmaa DA *et al.*:

Salvage radiotherapy for recurrent prostate cancer after radical prostatectomy. *JAMA.* 291: 1325-32, 2004.

[25] Katz MS, Zelefsky MJ, Venkatraman ES, Fuks Z, Hummer A and Leibel SA: Predictors of biochemical outcome with salvage conformal radiotherapy after radical prostatectomy for prostate cancer. *J. Clin. Oncol.* 21: 483-9, 2003.

[26] Moul JW, Wu H, Sun L, McLeod DG, Amling C, Donahue T, Kusuda L, Sexton W, O'Reilly K, Hernandez J *et al.*: Early versus delayed hormonal therapy for prostate specific antigen only recurrence of prostate cancer after radical prostatectomy. *J. Urol.* 171: 1141-7, 2004.

[27] Partin AW, Piantadosi S, Sanda MG, Epstein JI, Marshall FF, Mohler JL, Brendler CB, Walsh PC and Simons JW: Selection of men at high risk for disease recurrence for experimental adjuvant therapy following radical prostatectomy. *Urology.* 45: 831-8, 1995.

[28] D'Amico AV, Whittington R, Malkowicz SB, Fondurulia J, Chen MH, Tomaszewski JE and Wein A: The combination of preoperative prostate specific antigen and postoperative pathological findings to predict prostate specific antigen outcome in clinically localized prostate cancer. *J. Urol.* 160: 2096-101, 1998.

[29] Blute ML, Bergstralh EJ, Iocca A, Scherer B and Zincke H: Use of Gleason score, prostate specific antigen, seminal vesicle and margin status to predict biochemical failure after radical prostatectomy. *J. Urol.* 165: 119-25, 2001.

[30] Moul JW, Connelly RR, Lubeck DP, Bauer JJ, Sun L, Flanders SC, Grossfeld GD and Carroll PR: Predicting risk of prostate specific antigen recurrence after radical prostatectomy with the Center for Prostate Disease Research and Cancer of the Prostate Strategic Urologic Research Endeavor databases. *J. Urol.* 166: 1322-7, 2001.

[31] Freedland SJ, Terris MK, Csathy GS, Kane CJ, Amling CL, Presti JC, Jr., Dorey F and Aronson WJ: Preoperative model for predicting prostate specific antigen recurrence after radical prostatectomy using percent of biopsy tissue with cancer, biopsy Gleason grade and serum prostate specific antigen. *J. Urol.* 171: 2215-20, 2004.

In: Prostatectomies
Editors: H. Alvelos and Y. Izidoro
ISBN: 978-1- 62081-077-4
© 2012 Nova Science Publishers, Inc.

Chapter VI

Techniques for Neuro-Vascular Bundle Preservation

Christian I. Villeda Sandoval and Carlos E. Mendez Probst*

*Urology, Instituto Nacional de Ciencias Médicas y Nutrición "Salvador Zubirán" Mexico City, México

Abstract

Radical prostatectomy (RP) is the gold standard treatment for localized prostate cancer. Since excellent survival rates are reported with this therapeutic approach, functionality is the next major concern nowadays. Sexual potency is a mayor issue, so neuro-vascular bundle (NVB) preservation is the rule when indicated. Walsh published the first anatomical nerve-sparing technique for radical prostatectomy. He described detailed anatomy of the cavernous nerves and their distribution around the prostate. He also showed how to avoid neural injury by incising the lateral pelvic fascia anterior to the NVB and dividing the lateral pedicles closely to the prostate. Further improvements in the detail of the periprostatic neural anatomy have been accomplished. Anterior and posterior branches of the NVB have been defined, as well as the predominant NVB and accessory neural pathways. Finally, although the vast majority of nerves are found in the rectolateral sides of the prostate, a significant amount of nerve bundles are found in superior lateral portions.

Meticulous anatomy descriptions and technological advances such as surgical magnification (loupes), laparoscopy and robot assisted surgery have improved NVB preservation and different techniques have been described.

It is accepted that the NVB is located between the 2 layers of the lateral pelvic fascia (lateral levator fascia and medial prostatic fascia). The classical nerve-sparing technique in open RP states that the prostatic fascia must remain on the prostate. Minor modifications include a more anterior or superior initial incision to preserve more nerve branches. Laparoscopic and robot assisted methods share common technical steps. An intrafascial dissection plane between the prostate capsule and the prostatic fascia can be employed, as well as an interfascial plane between the prostatic fascia and the lateral pelvic fascia. An antegrade and a retrograde approach has also been described. Variations from the original descriptions, such as the "Veil of Aphrodite", athermal, clipless, traction-free or hydrodissection techniques have been reported. Hemostatic aids with different energy sources are commonly employed, but avoidance of its use during NVB dissection to prevent tissue damage is, currently, the preferred tactic. Novel techniques have been defined, such as ultrasound guidance, laser dissection or real-time augmented reality with neural or prostatic tissue identification. Their potential is being currently investigated. Potency outcomes with the open, laparoscopic or robot-assisted techniques have been published with comparable successful results.

Introduction

Despite recent advance in surgical technique and equipment, Retropubic Radical prostatectomy (RP) remains the gold standard for the treatment of organ-confined prostate cancer [1]. Neuro-vascular bundle (NVB) preservation in nerve-sparing RP introduced by Walsh [2] is the current treatment for localized disease, with acceptable post-operatory erectile function rates.

Laparoscopic and robotic-assisted laparoscopic surgery are the latest improvements in surgical armamentaria RP. In 1992, the first Laparoscopic RP was reported by Shuessler et al. [3], and Abbou et al. reported the first Robotically assisted laparoscopic RP in 2000 [4]. Many technical refinements have followed Walsh's improvement in open RP. Visual magnification in laparoscopic surgery or 3D vision and 360° precise movements in robotic-assisted surgery have further stimulated upgrades in the traditional technique.

Currently, open, laparoscopic and robotic-assisted RP offer excellent survival rates for organ-confined disease, functionality then is the next major item for the patient. Sexual potency being a major concern, so neuro-vascular bundle (NVB) preservation is of main interest for every urologist who performs RP. The following review summarizes the state of the art knowledge regarding this topic.

Neuro-Vascular Bundle Anatomical Considerations

The pelvic organs and external genitalia are innervated by the pelvic plexus. The parasympathetic visceral efferent preganglionic fibers arise from S2 to S4 in the sacral cord. The sympathetic fibers begin from T11 to L2 in the thoracolumbar region. The pelvic plexus provides innervation to the bladder, ureter, seminal vesicles, prostate, rectum, urethra and corpora cavernosa. The autonomic innervation to the corpora cavernosa is derived from the pudendal nerve and the pelvic plexus. The fibers to the corpora cavernosa travel outside the prostatic capsule [5] in association with the dorsolateral capsular arteries and veins of the prostate [6] (figure 1 and 2). Their location can be estimated by using accompanying capsular prostatic vessels as a landmark. The cavernosal nerves are contained in displaceable nerve bundles, located in the lateral pelvic fascia between the prostatic and the levator ani fascia[2, [7]].

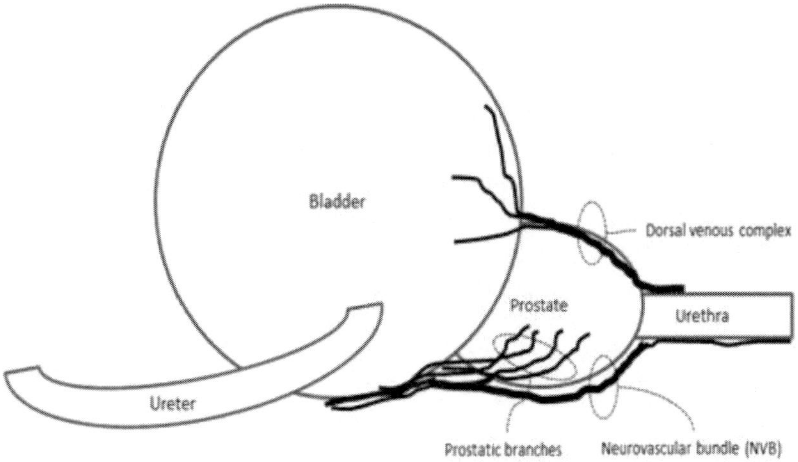

Figure 1. Neuro-vascular bundle anatomic relationship (lateral view).

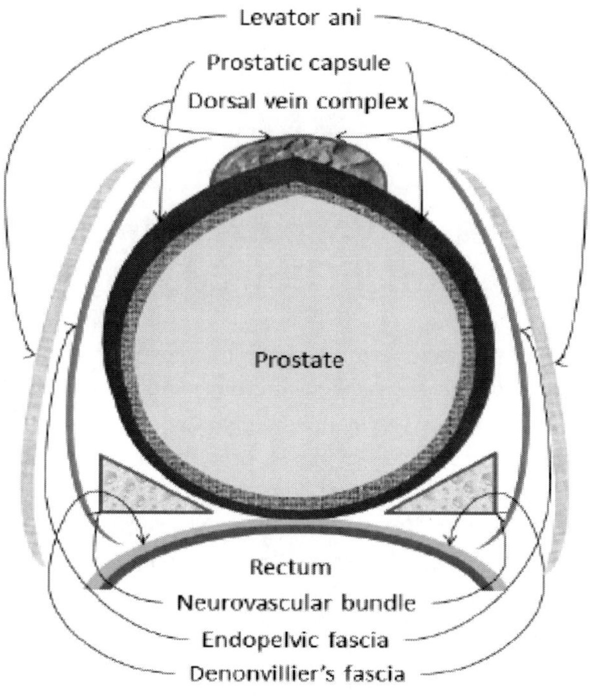

Figure 2. Neuro-vascular bundle anatomic relationship (coronal cross-section).

Anatomical Neuro-Vascular Bundle (NVB) Variants

Recent anatomical descriptions have shown that periprostatic nerves are not distributed entirely on the dorsolateral surface. Kyoshima et al. found that the classical NVB was only found in 48% of the prostates that they studied [8]. Furthermore, Eichelberg et al. located 45.9% to 65.6% of the nerves in the classical posterolateral location, in the 4 and 5, and 8 and 9 o'clock sectors of the prostate in a coronal plane.

Only 3 to 5% of the nerves were found near the rectal Denonviliier's fascia in the 6 and 7 o'clock sectors. However, 21.5% to 28.5% of the nerves were located in the 1 to 3, and 10 to 12 o'clock sectors (figure 3) [9]. Alsaid et al developed a 3D reconstruction of the nerve fibers surrounding the prostate of human male fetuses.

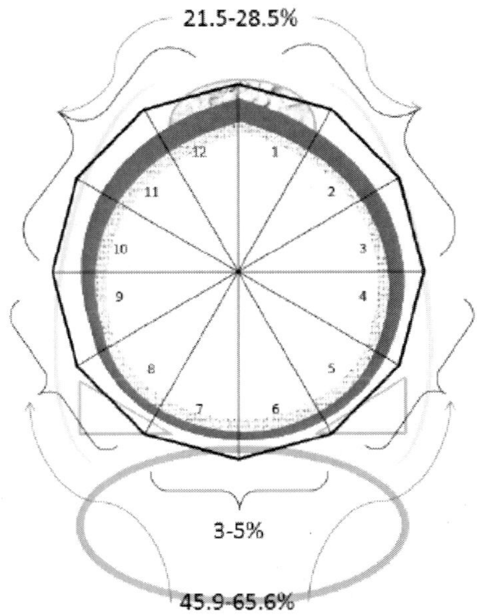

Figure 3. Clock sectors for Neuro-vascular bundle identification (coronal cross-section).

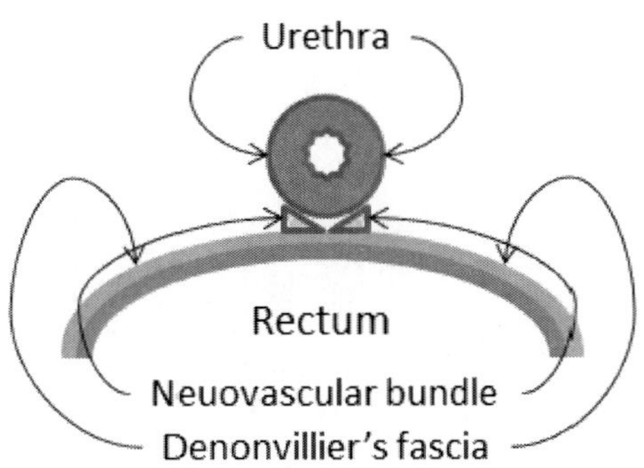

Figure 4. Neuro-vascular bundle adjacent to the urethra (coronal cross-section).

They found the existence of nerve fibers in the classical posterolateral position, but also in the anterolateral aspect, around the 11 to 2 o'clock sectors. Unfortunately they did not make an absolute count. They also demonstrated that the nerve fibers in the anterolateral aspect include sympathetic, parasympathetic and sensitive nerves [10]. Kaiho et al. performed intraoperative electric neuroestimulation of the lateral nerves on the surface on the prostate. They showed that the fibers between 1 and 5 o'clock sectors produced a raise in cavernosal pressure when stimulated. Nevertheless, the fibers in the 4 and 5 o´clock sectors had an increased effect [11]. A potential participation of these fibers in erectile function has not been directly demonstrated, but is strongly suspected.

Another important anatomical consideration is the location of the NVB after it leaves the prostate. The nerve fibers travel along the dorsolateral surface of the proximal urethra above the Denonvillier´s fascia [12] (figure 4).

Periprostatic Fascias and Preservation of the Neuro-Vascular Bundle (NVB)

The prostate is surrounded by a "prostatic capsule", which is a fibro-muscular tissue located between glandular units and periprostatic connective tissue, instead of a true capsule [13]. The endopelvic fascia covers the prostate and the bladder. It thickens and insert into the pubic bone as the puboprostatic ligaments. This fascia is considered to be composed of two distinct layers. The inner layer is considered as part of the Prostatic fascia and the outer layer as part of the Levator ani fascia (also called Lateral Pelvic fascia). The Dennonvilliers fascia covers the rectum posterior to the prostate.

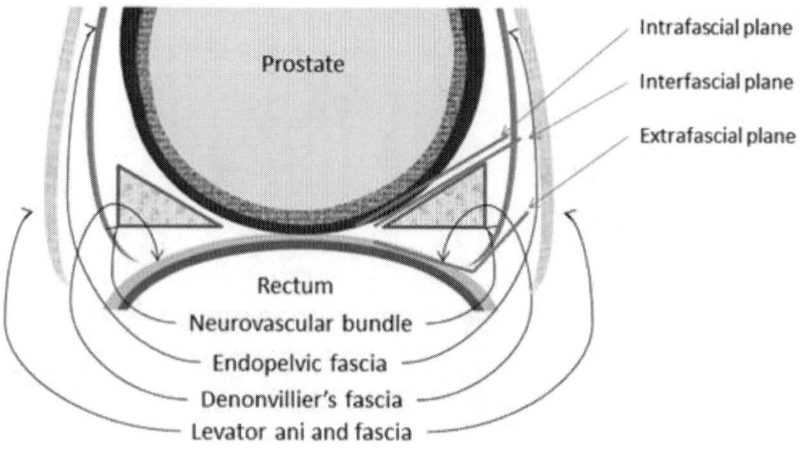

Figure 5. Fascial dissection planes.

Fascial plane knowledge is vital for successful NVB management. An intrafascial plane is the located between the prostate capsule and the prostatic fascia. The interfascial plane is created laterally between the prostatic fascia and the Levator ani fascia and ventrally, between the prostatic fascia and the Denonvillier's fascia. NVB preservation can be accomplished only by intrafascial or interfascial plane dissection [14] (figure 5).

Effects of Energy in Neuro-Vascular Bundle (NVB) Dissection

Thermal energy may directly affect unmyelinated nerve fibers. Thermal energy is therefore forbidden during NVB dissection. Ong et al. assessed the effect of hemostatic energy sources on the recovery of cavernous nerve function in a canine model. Exclusive suture ligation in the dissection without energy hemostatic sources had the best acute neural recovery rates. Both monopolar and bipolar energy caused decreased neural function, as well as the ultrasonic dissector [15]. Ahlering et al. confirmed the effect of thermal energy during NVB dissection in potency after surgery. They showed significant differences at two year follow-up with 63.2% of patients operated with cautery during dissection achieving functional penile erections in comparison to 92% of patients operated without thermal energy [16,17].

Gianduzzo et al. explored the feasibility of laser energy usage during NVB dissection. This group used a 1064 nm Nd:YAG laser to divide the tissue between the NVB and the prostatic fascia in combination with blunt dissection. Histological analysis measuring the depth of necrosis caused by the laser showed a 327 μm maximum depth of necrosis and 687 μm mean depth tissue injury [18]. They stated that minimum adjacent tissue injury was caused, although further evaluation is required.

Surgical Technique for Neuro-Vascular Bundle (NVB) Preservation

Walsh et al. published the first anatomical nerve-sparing technique for radical prostatectomy[2,5]. The NVB preservation must be planned. First, the endopelvic fascia is entered near the pelvic sidewall, well away from its attachment to the prostate and bladder, followed by dissection of the levator ani attachments to the level of the lateral pelvic fascia, then division of the puboprostatic ligaments and ligation of the dorsal vein complex. The urethra is cut over the Foley catheter with attention to the sphincter complex. Then, a plane is created between Denonvilliers' fascia and separated from the anterior wall of the rectum aided with gentle traction of the prostate with the Foley catheter.

At this point the course of the neurovascular bundle is usually visualized. Next, incision of the lateral fascia in an anterior point, in order to preserve the NVB in its posterolateral course (figure 6). The incision is extended cranially up to the area of the prostatic pedicle and once the lateral fascia is divided on both sides, the prostate can be separated from the rectum with the lateral pedicles divided close to the prostate in order to avoid injury to the NVB (figure 7). Several modifications to the classic technique for NVB preservation have been published. Lunacek et al. described a "curtain dissection" of the NVB [19]. They found that during fetal development, the fibers of the cavernosal nerves enclose the prostate and membranous urethra dorsally and laterally. During the growth of the prostate, the nerve fibers are anteriorly displaced and spread, forming a "curtain" around the prostate (figure 8).

They propose to start the dissection of the NVB further anteriorly, dissect the urethra, cut it and place the anastomotic sutures. Then, start the NVB dissection from the lateral and ventral aspect of the proximal urethra to the lateral pedicles, recommending to avoid the use of right-angle clamps during urethral dissection because nerve fibers run ventrally to the urethra (figure 4).

Masterson et al. [20]. have hypothesized that using traction to displace anteriorly and laterally the prostate during dissection may cause tension on the NVB resulting in possible traction injury. They propose a different approach in which before urethral division and mobilization of the prostate, the NVB is completely dissected off the prostate from the apex to a level above the seminal vesicles.

Additionally, Denonvilliers´ fascia is incised along the length of the prostate to further lateralize the NVB. After this modifications, the NVB is free of traction during the rest of the dissection and manipulation. They obtained an objective 22% improvement in erectile function at 6 months using this modifications.

Laparoscopic and robotic surgery have unique technical details when attempting NVB preservation. Magnification allows detailed anatomic dissections, but the reduced surgical field originates challenging procedural steps.

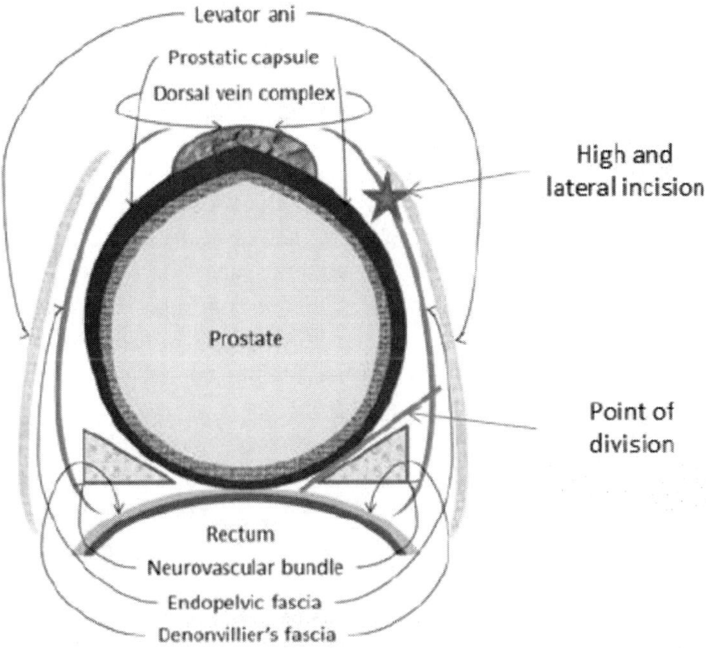

Figure 6. Classic incision and fascial plane dissection according to Walsh (coronal cross-section).

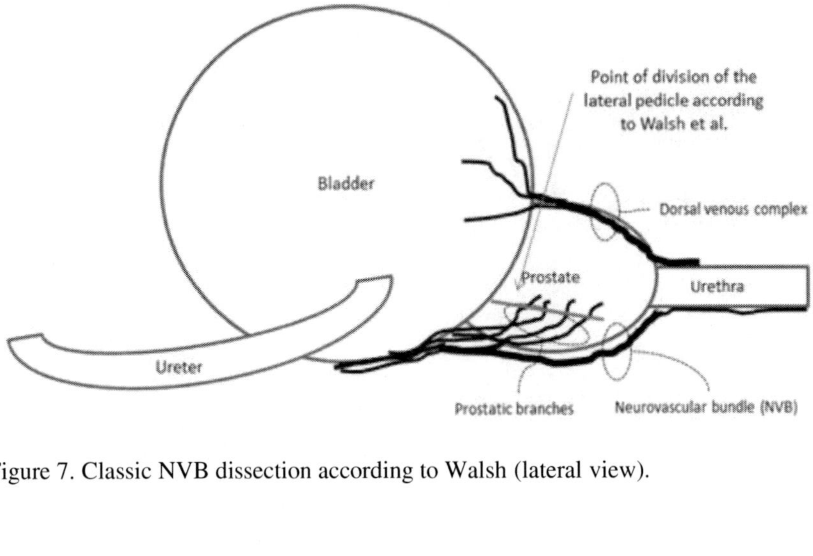

Figure 7. Classic NVB dissection according to Walsh (lateral view).

Laparoscopic radical prostatectomy has been described using two different approaches, the antegrade and the retrograde techniques [21,22,23,2425,26,27]. The retrograde technique includes the NVB dissection after controlling the dorsal vein complex and before division of the urethra. The levator ani fascia is incised anterolaterally from the base of the prostate to the apex, exposing the NVB.

The prostatic fascia is separated from the prostate. To detach the apex from the NVB, the plane between the two leaves of the lateral pelvic fascia is developed laterally to the prostatic urethral junction. However, the exact relationship of the NVBs and lateral pedicles cannot be identified optimally with this approach. Rassweiler et al. have proposed to use a complementary antegrade technique. The seminal vesicles and prostate are dissected before the proximal attachments of the NVB are liberated.

The antegrade technique mandates dissection of the seminal vesicles before approaching the NVB. Then the levator fascia is incised to develop a lateral NVB groove. After bladder neck division and lateral pedicle ligation, the lateral NVB groove is used as a guide for antegrade preservation of the NVB.

Both techniques avoid thermal energy and suture stitches at the 5 and 7 o'clock position in the urethra, to avoid NVB damage. Although the retrograde technique is more popular in open surgery, most laparoscopic urologists favor the antegrade approach because if offers prompt control of the prostatic pedicles and late division of the DVC compared with the retrograde approach. In experienced hands, there is no proven difference among both techniques regarding NVB preservation and postoperative sexual function [28].

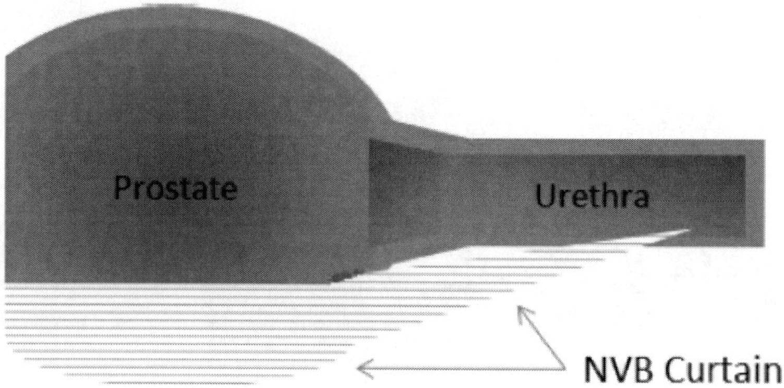

Figure 8. Curtain arrangement of nerve fibers (cranial view).

Laparoscopic and robot assisted methods share common tenants. An intrafascial dissection plane between the prostate capsule and the prostatic fascia has been employed, as well as an interfascial plane between the prostatic fascia and the lateral pelvic fascia.

Robot assisted surgery has several advantages over pure laparoscopic surgery. Three-dimensional vision, ergonomics and a broader angle movement arch have originated further modifications in the traditional laparoscopic technique. Athermal dissection is recommended as well as subtle traction14,28.

Menon et al.[29,30] have described the "veil of Aphrodite" technique for NVB preservation. Much like the previously described "curtain" dissection, based on the cavernosal nerve fibers extending from the posterolateral to the anterolateral surface of the prostate like a curtain (figure 8). With robot assistance, the interfascial plane between the posterior prostatic fascia and the Denonvillier's fascia is extended as distally as possible towards the apex. The pedicles are exposed and divided with clips or bipolar energy. Then the prostatic fascia is incised to create an intrafascial plane. The fascia is dissected off the prostate and is left hanging as a veil from the pubo-urethral ligaments. Histological and functional improvement has been demonstrated with this technique [31,32].

To further improvement in NVB preservation, avoidance of thermal coagulation energy, clips for hemostasis and even avoidance of countertraction have been described.

Kowalczyk et al. [33]. advocate to avoid any traction assistance when dissection the NVB away from the prostate. They used a combination of sharp and blunt dissection for the NVB and clips for pedicle ligation. They report improved potency at 5 months favoring dissection without countertraction, however, there was no difference at 12 months follow-up.

Clipless and athermal dissection have been individually used for nerve-sparing robotic-assisted radical prostatectomy [34,35]. Ahlering et al. described a combined approach where vascular clamps and sutures were used for pedicle control in order to give augmented protection to the NVB from mechanical and thermal trauma. Their group showed improved erectile function results, reaching 93% adequate erections at 2 years follow-up.

Guru et al. [36] published a simple innovative technique where hydrodissection of the neurovascular bundle was performed by injecting a 1:10000 epinephrine solution diluted in 0.9% normal saline into the lateral prostatic pedicle. He explained that this dissection aid allows a faster and safer dissection, although erectile function results are pending.

Real time intraoperative monitorization is the next step in preserving NVB during dissection. Rais-Bahrami et al. [37] used the Optical Coherence Tomography to identify cavernosal nerves in live rats and then used ex-vivo human prostates for the same analysis. This technique measures backscatter near-infrared light rather than sound, obtaining images of tissues with resolutions several orders of magnitude greater. They were able to identify cavernosal nerve fibers as hyperdense, linear structures. They suggest that real time usage of this technique may be the last frontier to conquer in order to preserve all NVB fibers.

References

[1] Bill-Axelson, A., Holmberg, L., Ruutu, M., Häggman, M., Andersson, S. O., Bratell, S. et al. Radical prostatectomy versus watchful waiting in early prostate cancer. *NEng. J. Med.* 2005;352:1977-84.

[2] Walsh, P. C., Donker, P. J. Impotence following radical prostatectomy: Insight into etiology and prevention. *J. Urol.* 1982;128:492-97.

[3] Schuessler, W. W., Schulam, P. G., Clauman, R. V., Kavoussi, L. R. Laparoscopic radical prostatectomy: initial shorterm experience. *Uroogy*. 1997; 50:854-7.

[4] Abbou, C. C., Hoznek, A., Salomon, L., Lobontiu, A., Saint, F., Cicco, A., Antiphon, P., Chopin, D. [Remote laparoscopic radical prostatectomy carried out with a robot. Report of a case]. *Prog. Urol.* 2000 Sep.;10(4):520-3. French.

[5] Walsh, P. C., Lepor, H., Eggleston, J. C. Radical prostatectomy with preservation of sexual function: anastomical and pathological considerations. *Prostate*. 1983;4;473-85.

[6] Walsh, P. C. Anatomic radical prostatectomy: evolution of the surgical technique. *J. Urol.* 1998; 160(6 Pt 2):2418-24.

[7] Lepor, H., Gregerman, M., Crosby, R., Mostofi, F. K., Walsh, P. C. Precise location of the autonomic nerves from the pelvic plexus to the corpora cavernosa: a detailed anatomical study of the adult male pelvis. *J. Urol.* 1985;144:207-12.

[8] Kyoshima, K., Yokomizo, A., Yoshida, T., Tomita, K., Yonemasu, H., Nakamura, M. et al. Anatomical features of periprostatic tissue and its surroundigs: a histological analysis of 79 radical retropubic prostatectomy specimens. *Jpn. J. Clin. Oncol*. 2004;34:463.

[9] Eichelberg, C., Erbersdobler, A., Michl, U., Schlomm, T., Salomon, G., Graefen, M., Huland, H. Nerve distribution along the prostatic capsule. *Eur. Urol.* 2007;51:105-11.

[10] Alsaid, B., Karam, I., Bessede, T., Abdlsamad, I., Uhl, J. F., Delmas, V., Benoît, G., Droupy, S. Tridimensional computer-assisted anatomic dissection of posterolateral prostatic neuravscular bundles. *Eur. Urol.* 2010;58:281-287.

[11] Kaiho, Y., Nakagawa, H., Saito, H., Ito, A., Ishidoya, S., Saito, S., Arai, Y. Nerves at the ventral prostatic capsule contribute to erectile function: initial electrophysiological assessment in humans. *Eur. Urol.* 2008;

[12] Lunacek, A., Schwentner, C., Fritsch, H., Bartsch, G., Strasser, H. Anatomical radical retropubic prostatectomy: 'curtain dissection' of the neurovascular bundle. *BJU Int.* 2005;95:1226-31.

[13] Ayala, A. G., Ro, J. Y., Babaian, R., Troncoso, P., Grignon, D. J. The prostatic capsule: does it exist? Its importance in the staging and treatment of prostatic carcinoma. *Am. J. Surg. Pathol.* 1989;13:21-7.

[14] Chauhan, S., Coelho, R. F., Rocco, B., Palmer, K. J., Orvieto, M. A., Patel, V. R. Techniques of nerve-sparing and potency outcomes following robot-assisted laparoscopic prostatectomy. *Int. Braz. J. Urol.* 2010;36(3):159-72.

[15] Nerve sparing radical prostatectomy: Effects of mhemostatic energy sources on the recovery of cavernous nerve function in a canine model. *J. Urol.* 2004;172:1318-22.

[16] Ahlering, T. E., Eichel, L., Skarecky, D. Early potency outcomes with cautery-free neurovascular bundle preservation with robotic laparoscopic radical prostatectomy. *J. Endourol.* 2005;19(6):715-18.

[17] Ahlering, T. E., Rodríguez, E., Skarecky, D. W. Overcoming obstacles: nerve-sparing issues in radical prostatectomy. *J. Endourol.* 2008;22: 745-50.

[18] Gianduzzo, T. R. J., Chang, C. M., El-Shazly, M., Mustajab, A., Moon, D. A., Eden, C. G. Laser nerve-sparing laparoscopic radical prostatectomy: a feasibility study. *BJU Int.* 2007;99:875-79.

[19] Lunacek, A., Schwentner, C., Fritsch, H., Bartsch, G., Strasser, H. Anatomical radical retropubic prostatectomy: 'curtain dissection' of the neurovascular bundle. *BJU Int.* 2005;95:1226-31.

[20] Masterson, T. A., Serio, A. M., Mulhall, J. P., Vickers, A. J., Eastham, J. A. Modified technique for neurovascular bundle preservation during radical prostatectomy: association between technique and recovery of erectile function. *BJU Int.* 2008;101:1217-22.

[21] Guillonneau, B., Vallancien, G. Laparoscopic radical prostatectomy: the Montsouris technique. *J. Urol.* 2000;163:1643-49.

[22] Rhee, H. K., Triaca, V., Sorcini, A., Tuerk, I. A. Transperitoneal laparoscopic radical prostatectomy: descending technique. *J. Endourol.* 2004;18:601-4.

[23] Su, L. M., Link, R. E., Bhayani, S. B., Sullivan, W., Pavlovich, C. P. Nerve-sparing laparoscopic radical prostatectomy: replicating the open surgical technique. *Urology.* 2004;64:123-7.

[24] Gill, I. S., Okimura, O., Rubinstein, M., Finelli, A., Moinzadeh, A., Singh, D., Kaouk, J., Miki, T., Desai, M. Lateral pedicle control during laparoscopic radical prostatectomy: refined technique. *Urology.* 2005;65: 23-7.

[25] Rassweiler, J. J., Sugiono, M., Hruza, M., Tefekli, A., Stock, C,. Teber, D. Retrograde nerve-sparing (NS) laparoscopic radical prostatectomy (LRP): Technical aspects and early results. *Eur. Urol.* 2006;5:925-33.

[26] Curto, F., Beijts, J., Pansadoro, A., Barmoshe, S., Hoepffner, J. L., Mugnier, C., Piechaud, T., Gaston, R. Nerve sparing laparoscopic radical prostatectomy: Our technique. *Eur. Urol.* 2006;49:344-52.

[27] Rassweiler, J. J., Hruza, M., Frede, T., Teber, D. Laparoscopic extraperitoneal ascending nerve-sparing radical prostatectomy: An effective and safe technique for apical tumors. *J. Endourol.* 2008;22(9):2009-13.

[28] Rassweiler, J. J., Wagner, A. A., Moazin, M., Gözen, A. S., Teber, D., Frede, T., Su, L. M. Anatomic nerve-sparing laparoscopic radical prostatectomy: comparison of retrograde and antegrade techniques. *Urology.* 2006;68(3):587-91.

[29] Menon, M., Tewari, A., PEabodly J. Vattikuti Institute prostatectomy: technique. *J. Urol.* 2003;169:2289-92.

[30] Kaul, S., Bhandari, A., Hemal, A., Savera, A., Shrivastava, A., Menon, M. Robotic radical prostatectomy with preservation of the prostatic fascia: a feasibility study. *Urology.* 2005;66:1261-5.

[31] Menon, M., Shrivastava, A., Kaul, S., Badani, K. K., Fumo, M., Bhandari, M., Peabody, J. O. Vittikuti Institute prostatectomy: contemporary technique and analysis of results. *Eur. Urol.* 2007;51: 648-57.

[32] Savera, A. T., Kaul, S., Badani, K., Stark, A. T., Sha, N. L., Menon, M. Robot radical prostatectomy with the "Veil of Aphrodite" technique: Histologic evidence of enhanced nerve sparing. *Eur. Urol.* 2006;49:1065-74.

[33] Kowalczyk, K. J., Huang, A. C., Hevelone, N. D., Lipsitz, S. R., Yu, H. Y., Ulmer, W. D., Kaplan, J. R., Patel, S., Nguyen, P. L., Hu, J. C. Stepwise approach for nerve sparing without countertraction during robot-assisted radical prostatectomy: technique and outcomes. *Eur. Urol.* 2011;60(3):536-47.

[34] Chien, G. W., Mikhail, A. A., Orvieto, M. A., Zagaja, G. P., Sokoloff, M. H., Brendler, C. B., Shalhav, A. L. Modified clipless antegrade nerve preservation in robotic-assisted laparoscopic radical prostatectomy with validated sexual function evaluation. *Urology*. 2005;66(2):419-23.

[35] Leung, R. A., Kim, T. S., Tewari, A. K. Future directions of robotic surgery: a case study of the Cornell athermal robotic technique of prostatectomy. *Scientific World Journal*. 2006;19(6):2553-9.

[36] Guru, K. A., Perlmutter, A. E., Butt, Z. M., Peabody, J. O. Hydrodissection for preservation of neurovascular bundle during robot-assisted radical prostatectomy. *Can. J. Urol.* 2008;15(2):4000-3.

[37] Rais-Bahrami, S., Levinson, A. W., Fried, N. M., Lagoda, G. A., Hristov, A., Chuang, Y., Burnett, A. L., Su, L. M. Optical coherence tomography of cavernous nerves: a step toward real-time intraoperative imaging during nerve-sparing radical prostatectomy. *Urology*. 2008;72(1):198-204.

In: Prostatectomies
Editors: H. Alvelos and Y. Izidoro
ISBN: 978-1- 62081-077-4
© 2012 Nova Science Publishers, Inc.

Chapter VII

Extraperitoneal Endoscopic Radical Prostatectomy: Techniques and Results*

Marcos Tobias-Machado[1,2,3], Eduardo S. Starling[1,2], Fernando Korkes[1], Ricardo L. Machado[2] and Eric R. Wroclawski[1,2,3]
[1]ABC Medical School, Sao Paulo, Brazil
[2]Brazilian Institute of Cancer Control (IBCC), Sao Paulo, Brazil
[3]Albert Einstein Jewish Hospital, Sao Paulo, Brazil

Abstract

Laparoscopic and robotic assisted radical prostatectomies are continuous developing techniques, with feasibility and reproducibility demonstrated worldwide. Low morbidity and excellent functional and oncological outcomes can be achieved, although learning curve without robotic assistance is longer. The majority of centers that employ this technique have preferred transperitoneal access. Few groups prefer endoscopic extra peritoneal route but this surgical access is currently

* A version of this chapter also appears in *New Cancer Research Developments*, edited by Thomas D. Ford, published by Nova Science Publishers, Inc. It was submitted for appropriate modifications in an effort to encourage wider dissemination of research.

receiving a higher acceptance. We herein review the improvements in our personal technique reporting current experience with endoscopic extra peritoneal radical prostatectomy (EEERP) as a first line therapy for localized prostate cancer.

In a 5-year period 120 patients underwent 5 to 6-port EEERP at our center in Brazil. Nerve sparing procedure was applied in 85% of surgeries, with mean operative time of 180 minutes after the 40 initial cases, and mean blood loss of 210 mL (transfusion rate 2.2%). Peritoneum perforation occurred in 40% and no conversion to open surgery was required. Complications occurred in 12.5% of men and median hospital stay was 2 days. Mean return to normal activities was 4 weeks. Erection sufficient to penetration in previous potent patients occurred in 75% of men and 98% of men remained continent. Overall positive surgical margin occurred in 10% and after a mean 3.5-year follow-up 90% of men were free of PSA recurrence.

EEERP can be performed with efficacy providing the benefits of both laparoscopy and a totally extra peritoneal approach. Severe complications related to learning curve (urinary and rectal fistula) seem to be less morbid in EEERP. Reduction of complication rate and better oncological and functional results can be achieved by surgeon experience, and robotic assistance might reduce the learning curve. An analysis of the literature shows equivalence between trans and extra peritoneal access in experienced hands. Reduced learning curve period favored robotic assisted surgery to introduce laparoscopic radical prostatectomy in USA. Costs, availability and training facilities are important issues related to acceptance of minimally invasive surgery in development countries.

Introduction

Surgical treatment for localized prostate cancer has proved to be an excellent treatment option, mainly concerning oncological outcomes and peroperative morbidity [1]. Currently three different approaches have been used: open, laparoscopic and robotic. Retropubic radical prostatectomy remains the most performed operation due to a large accumulated experience and long term follow up of large series of patients. However, a new dawn has emerged with novel minimally invasive modalities available, including both minimally invasive prostatectomy as well as newer energy sources as high-intensity focused ultrasound and cryotherapy. The ultimate goals of such novel minimally invasive modalities are to improve functional outcomes without compromising oncological results.

Extraperitoneal (EP) endoscopic radical prostatectomy combines the advantages of EP surgery and those of minimally invasive techniques. This review summarizes data available about EP endoscopic radical prostatectomy, in terms of technique, oncological and functional outcomes.

Radical Prostatectomt: Surgical Approachs

Traditionally, the best initial treatment for men with prostate cancer who had a predictable survival of more than 10 years had been open radical prostatectomy. However, over the last 10 years, laparoscopic radical prostatectomy (LRP) has become more accepted worldwide. Very recently, robot-assisted techniques have emerged as a viable option mainly for surgeons without special skills in laparoscopic surgery, challenging the other approaches. The role of minimally invasive techniques in the evolving field of prostate cancer management is yet to be determined, and is the subject of the present review.

Because of the anatomic topography of the prostate gland, radical prostatectomy has been a difficult operation to perform with the potential for significant adverse side effects. Therefore, over the years, simpler means of treating patients with prostate cancer have been sought. Young described radical prostatectomy in 1905 for treating men with localized prostate cancer [2]. In 1982, Walsh introduced a reformulated technique for performing radical retropubic prostatectomy, which brought the possibility of preserving urinary continence and erections, and lowering mortality rates to 0-0.4% [1,3]. Subsequent refinements made radical prostatectomy even safer and more effective [1,4,5].

Schuessler introduced laparoscopic approach to prostate cancer surgery in 1992 [6]. In this initial report LRP was characterized as an "extensively long and difficult operation without advantages when compared to the open approach" [6]. LRP remained considered experimental until further feasibility and reproducibility were proved [7]. Larger European series have subsequently been reported in France and Germany proving that LRP was not only feasible but also as efficient and safe as the open approach [8]. The advantages of this minimally invasive surgery were than brought to the forefront, increasing the appeal of such procedures for both patients and surgeons. The combination of improved cosmetics, shorter convalescence, decreased morbidity and improvement in surgical efficiency led to increased patient demand. Since than, many urologists have adopted the LRP technique. Early experiences with LRP were performed through transperitoneal (TP) approach. In 1998, Guillonneau et al. introduced the technique of antegrade laparoscopic radical prostatectomy through TP access, which was subsequently reproduced by other services [9]. According to the authors, the initial access to the seminal vesicles prior to the dorsal vein complex ligation were essential technical modifications that made the LRP easier. Rassweiller et al. introduced LRP with antegrade prostatic dissection and approaching the seminal vesicles through the posterior bladder neck (Heinbronn technique) [10]. Raboy et al. first described EP-LRP [11]. Except for the initial dissection of seminal vesicles, they employed the French technique, sectioning the venous complex and the urethra as the final steps of prostatic ablation. Dubernard et al. described the first series of retrograde EP-LRP, demonstrating the excellent outcomes with the method [12]. In Brazil, laparoscopic radical prostatectomy has been performed in a few centers, mostly through TP route. Our personal impression is that TP and EP techniques have similar surgical time, blood loss, complications and post-operative recovery period.

Table 1. Laparoscopic instruments and surgical matherials

0 o laparoscope
High flow insufflators
2 10/12mm trocars
4 5mm trocars
Fine dissecting scissors
Fine grasping forceps
Fenestrated grasping forceps
Ultrasonic scalpel
Bipolar cauterizing grasper
Metallic urethral sound (Beniquet forceps) with a divot at the end 18Fr.11) 2
Needle holders
Titanium clip applier
Purple Hem-O-lock applier
Irrigation and suction tube
Endocatch bag R
Silicon Foley catheter 20Fr
Penrose drain no 2
3 Vicryl 2-0, CT needle (37mm)
2 Monocryl 3-0 (26mm) needle

As original contributions we have performed retrograde dissection as described in the open technique, employing a polymer clip that helps to avoid venous reflux from the dorsal vein complex, and also aids in the subsequent identification of the bladder neck.

External handling and sectioning of the Foley catheter enables internal and superior traction by the assistant, as in the open technique, which helps to access the posterior aspect of the prostate. Such dissection helps to identify the lateral prostatic pedicles following the dissection of the bladder neck. The accurate identification of the prostatic contour is fundamental not only for a proper identification of the neurovascular bundles but also to avoid the occurrence of positive margins [13].

More recently we have used the EP antegrade technique as described for the Heinbronn technique, sectioning the dorsal vein complex and the urethra as the final step of prostate ablation [14].

The advent of the Da Vinci system to assist laparoscopic surgery served as a platform to enhance surgeons' skills and to define further technological advantages, such as better 3D vision and the development of "wrist" articulated instruments that maintain tactic perception. In 2001, approximately 250 robotic-assisted laparoscopic prostatectomies (RALP) were performed; in 2007, this number was estimated in over 50,000 surgeries [15].

This new technology has the potential to equip the urologist with microsurgical precision that can help to improve functional results without compromising oncological outcomes.

Radical Prostatectomy: Comparative Outcomes of Different Approachs

Complications and Effectiveness

The open surgery has become the gold standard reference for all comparisons. Large contemporary series of patients treated with open radical prostatectomy with up to 15-year-follow up are available [1, 16]. In a large series with seven-year-follow up overall survival rate was 90% and the cancer-specific survival rate was 97% (i.e., only 3% of patients died of prostate cancer within seven years of surgery) [17]. This cancer-specific survival rate is consistent with the results reported from other contemporary radical prostatectomy series [1, 15]

Operative Time

The surgical time has been a sticking point of the minimally invasive approach, both laparoscopic and robotic. The initial operative time of laparoscopic surgeries were tremendously long [18] but were improving as learning curves advanced [19].

With robotic surgery operative time is also shortening significantly as experience increase. Operative time in the initial RALP learning curve seems to be something inferior to LRP and very similar to operative-time of open prostatectomy reported in recent series.

Blood Loss

Blood loss is significantly reduced during LRP or RALP, thereby decreasing blood transfusion rates. A pressure of 1215 mmHg helps to tamponate small oozing vessels, which are generally responsible for bleeding during open prostatectomy. Most series report losses below 100-200 ml [20].

Postoperative Pain

Comparative studies about postoperative pain demonstrate a clear benefit for laparoscopic vs. open approach [21].

Urinary Continence

Surgical technique is directly associated with the occurrence of stress urinary incontinence after radical prostatectomy. Intrinsic sphincteric deficiency is common in the first weeks, but the vast majority of patients recover continence after several weeks [22].

Distinctive methods for evaluation urinary incontinence rates reported (questionnaires, personal interview, telephone contact, etc.), incontinence definition and classification, make very difficult to establish objective comparisons. To the present date, there is no evidence to assert that an approach is associated with better continence outcomes when compared to the others.

Sexual Function

It is unquestionable that dissection principles of the neurovascular bundles must be the same regardless of techniques or approaches employed. After EP-LRP with clear use of electrocoagulation Stolzenburg et al. reported 12% of patients with sufficient erection for intercourse after unilateral NS and a 47% after bilateral NS (s after 6-month-follow up, with IPDE5) [23,24].

Potency rates have been reported varying from had a 43-76% for LRP with bilateral NS procedures after a 12month-follow up [25,26].

Oncological Follow-up

After more than 15 years, open radical prostatectomy has demonstrated excellent oncological results [27], whereas data is still limited for LRP and RALP.

In the Mayo Clinic open surgery series, biochemical success rate for 3 and 5 years were 99% and 98% respectively [28].

Guillonneau et al., obtained a biochemical success rate after 1,000 procedures of 92%, 88%, 77% and 44% for pT2a, pT2b, pT3a and pT3b respectively [29]. Rozet et al. have recently published biochemical success rates of 95% after 12 months of follow up [26].

While no series with sufficiently long follow up are available to analyze oncological outcomes, possible surrogate parameters are evaluated. In such context, positive surgical margins have been compared after radical prostatectomy and the three approaches seem to be equally effective to eradicate local disease, and a longer follow up is necessary to allow further comparisons.

Endoscopic Extraperitoneal Radical Prostatectomy

The TP approach is the conventional technique for LRP. There are however several disadvantages of this approach, such as a higher risk of injury to intraperitoneal organs and longer postoperative ileum. To prevent these complications, we have adopted EP approach, similar to open radical prostatectomy [30].

EP-LRP technique can be performed by antegrade or retrograde dissection. The antegrade one is performed from the bladder neck to the prostate apex [11]. Our EP technique is described below. We have performed it since 2002 duplicating open surgery's steps, but sectioning the dorsal vein complex and the urethra at the end of prostatic ablation.

In the last 5 years, we have performed over 150 five to six-port LRP at our institution. The initial protocol included patients with low volume, low grade and low body mass index. After 50 cases no exclusion criteria were further adopted.

Instrumentation

Basic instrumentation is the same for all EP laparoscopic surgeries in our center. In our experience the bipolar or harmonic and fenestrated grasping forceps are very important instruments to achieve a success exposition and traction to control of the vessels.

Surgical Steps of Retrograde Technique

1. Patient is placed in horizontal dorsal decubitus, abducting the lower limbs with a light Trendelemburg position (Figure 1);
2. Display of the surgical team: The surgeon operates on the left side, the camera is positioned at the upper end of the table, and the assistant stand at the patient's right side. During suture, for improved comfort, the surgeon and the camera switch places? (Figure 1);
3. Umbilical incision measuring 1.5 cm up to the Retzius space;
4. Creation of extraperitoneal space through digital dissection and manufactured or homemade balloon dilator ();
5. Hasson trocar (10 mm) through the umbilical incision for the 0-degrees optic;
6. Installation of pneumoretroperitonium with 15 mmHg CO_2 tension;
7. Introduction of 4 working trocars (2 external pararectal measuring 10 mm, and 2 in the iliac fossa measuring 5 mm) under direct view, in an arciform shape, with caution to avoid peritoneal lesion . In selected cases a 6th suprapubic trocar is necessary for retraction to aid better exposition (Figure 3);

8. Exeresis of pre-prostatic fat with monopolar cautery to identify the prostate, bladder, endopelvic fascia and puboprostatic ligaments (Figure 4);
9. Bilateral opening of endopelvic fascia with scissors, while performing contralateral traction of the prostate (Figure 5);
10. Identification and section of puboprostatic ligaments;

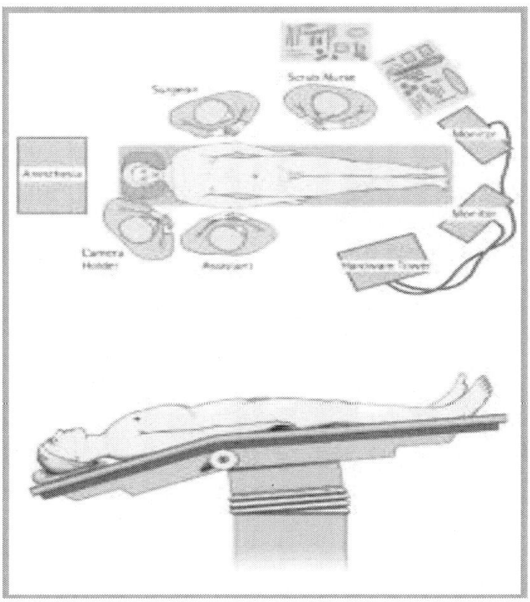

Figure 1. Patient and surgical team position.

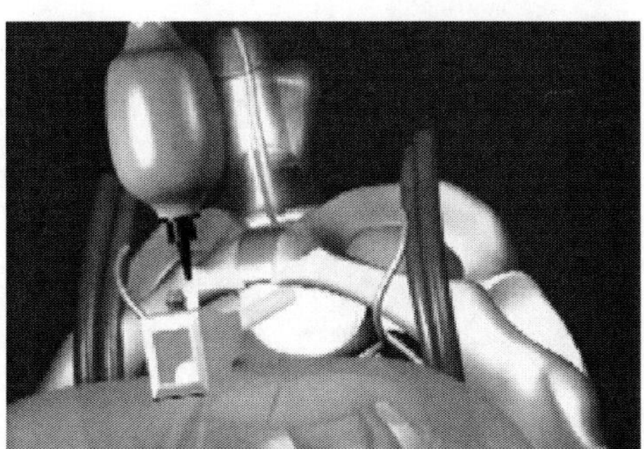

Figure 2. Preperitoneal balloon insuflation.

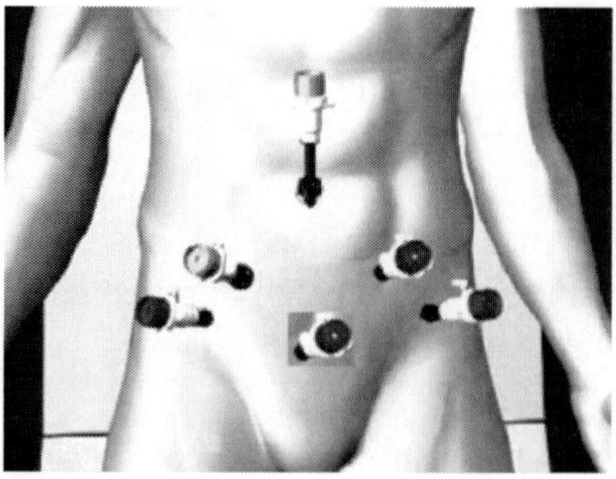

Figure 3. Trocar placement.

a

b

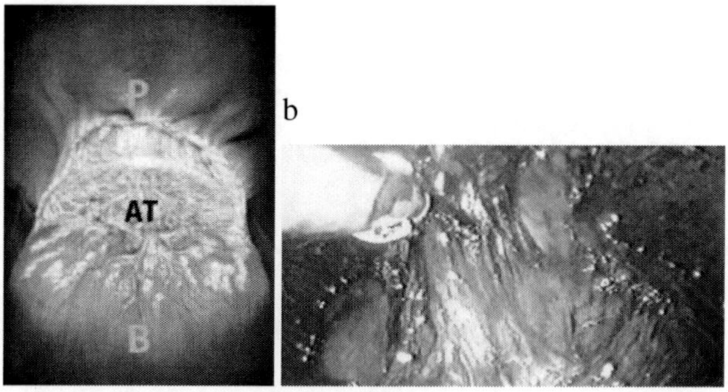

Figure 4. Exeresis of pre-prostatic fat with monopolar cautery (schematic and endoscopic view). P – Pubic bone; AT- Adipose tissue; B- Bladder.

A

B

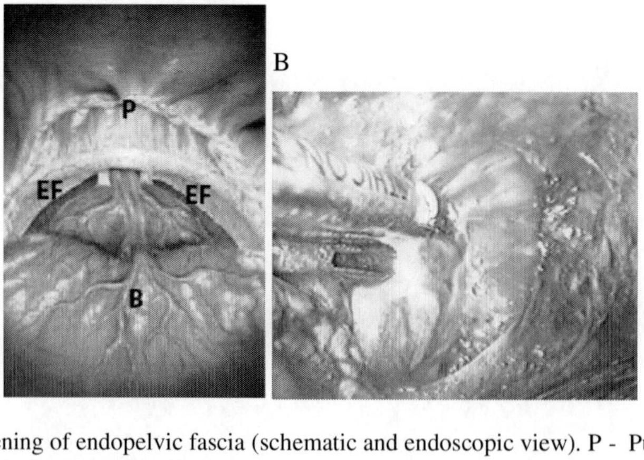

Figure 5. Opening of endopelvic fascia (schematic and endoscopic view). P - Pubic bone; EF- Endopelvic fascia;B - Bladder.

a

b

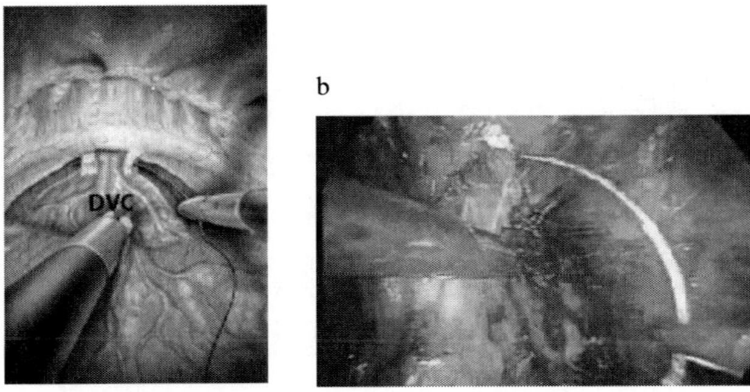

DVC- Dorsal vein complex

Figure 6. Vascular control of dorsal vein complex (schematic and endoscopic view).

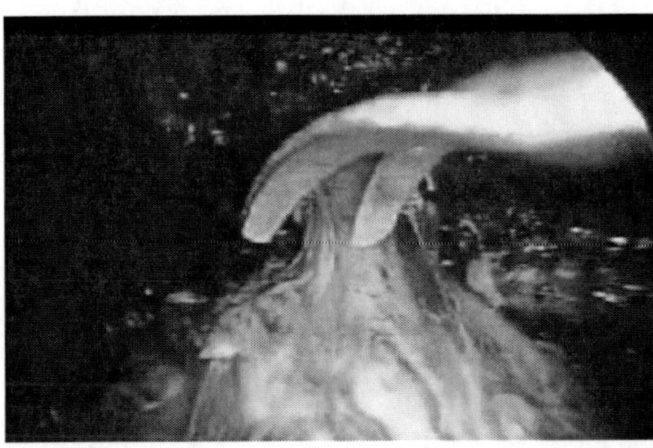

Figure 7. Apical dissection with scissors.

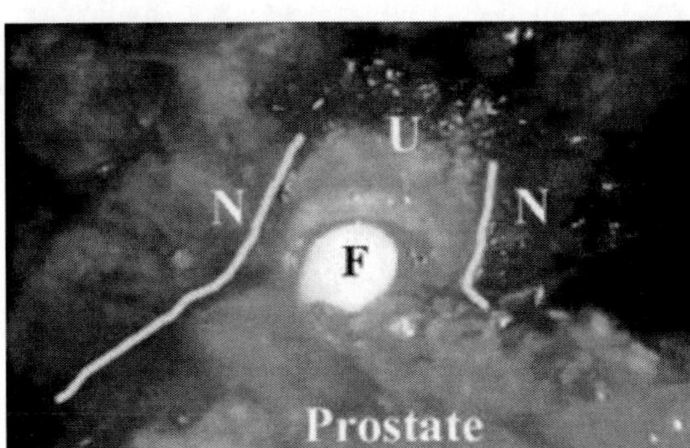

Figure 8. Open the urethra protecting the neurovascular bundles [13]. U-Urethra; N - Neurovascular bundles; F – Foley catheter.

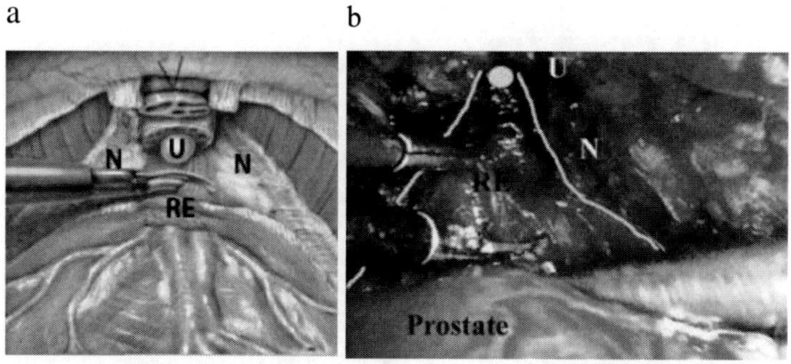

Figure 9. Retroprostatic dissection (schematic and endoscopic view). N – Neurovascular bundle; U – Urethra; RE- Retroprostatic space.

11. Dorsal vein complex control with a "X" stitch using 2-0 polyglactine suture with CT-1 needle (Figure 6) and control of the retrograde blood flow with harmonic scalpel, bipolar scalpel or polymer clip (Hem-o-lockÆ). Applying the clip makes the subsequent identification of the bladder neck easier for reconstruction, a surgical step that is often arduous when we choose to preserve the bladder neck;
12. Apical dissection preserving the sphincteric apparatus (figure 7);
13. Sectioning the dorsal vein complex with electrocautery or harmonic scalpel, until the urethra is viewed;
14. Opening anterior urethral wall with scissors (Figure 8). Section is performed after perfectly identifying the limits of the prostate apex and urethra, thus avoiding positive margins;
15. The balloon is filled with 20 mL of distilled water. The Foley catheter is externally pulled for subsequent knot application with 0-cotton suture including both drainage and balloon routes;
16. Sectioning of the catheter close to the previously applied knot;
17. Recovery of the remaining stump of the Foley catheter, through endoscopic view in the extraperitoneal space;
18. Posterior section of the urethra and recto-urethralis muscle following cranial traction of the stent by the assistant;
19. Blunt retroprostatic dissection up to the most proximal point as possible (figure 9);
20. Identification and opening of the posterior layer of the Dennovilliers fascia. At this point it is possible to identify the pre-rectal fat. As in open surgery, we know that the neurovascular bundle lies laterally and

under the fascia, which makes nervous preservation easier while ligating the prostatic pedicle, which is performed by posterior access;

21. Sectioning the bladder neck, preserving muscular fibers whenever possible. The dissection is started with harmonic or bipolar scalpel and upon reaching the urethral mucosa, it is sectioned with scissors (Figure 10);
22. Identification of correct plane between posterior bladder neck and posterior prostate to identify vasa deferentia and seminal vesicles;
23. Dissection and division of vasa deferentia with harmonic or monopolar scalpel;
24. Superior traction of the vasa deferentia by the assistant in order to easy release the seminal vesicles. At this time, we preferred to use harmonic or bipolar scalpel in order to avoid dissipation of thermal energy that could damage the nervi erigentes;

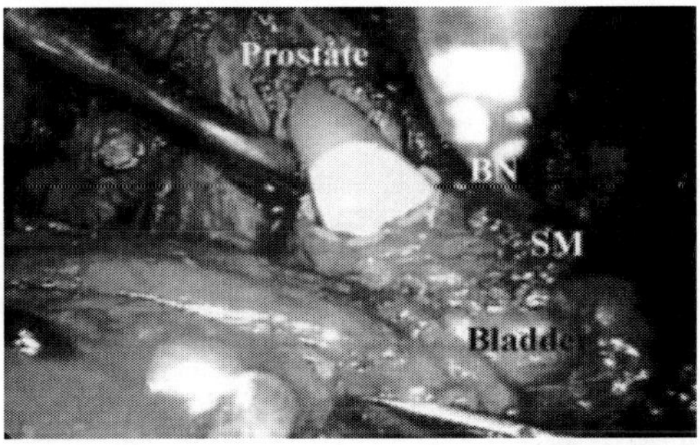

Figure 10. Dissection with preservation of the bladder neck [13]. BN- Bladder neck; SM- Smooth muscle.

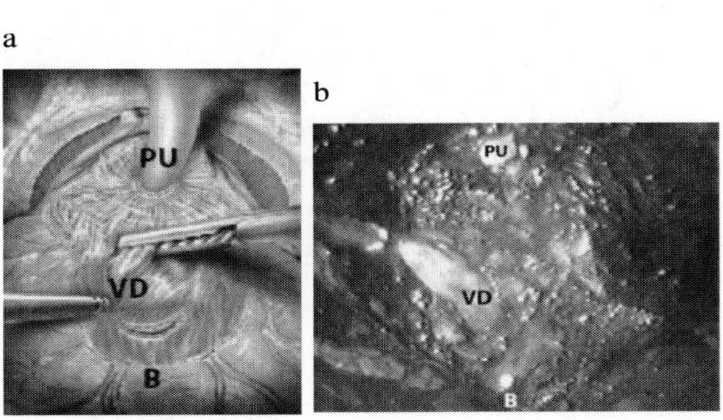

Figure 11. Dissection of vasa deferens (schematic and endoscopic view). PU- Prostatic urethra; VD- Vasa deferens; B – Bladder.

a b

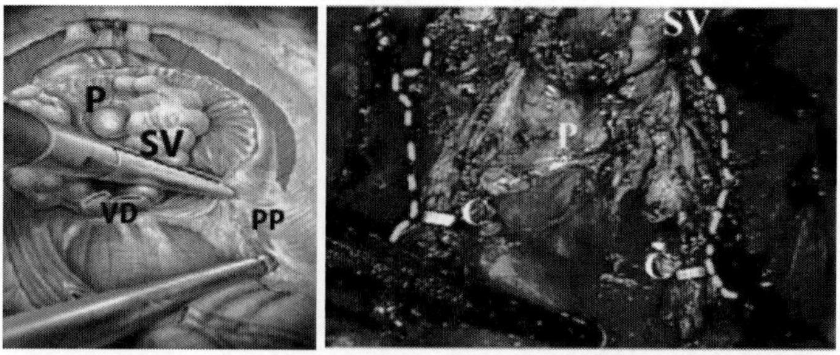

Figure 12. The prostatic pedicles are identified and clipped [13] (schematic and endoscopic view). P- Prostate; VD- Vasa deferens; PP – Prostatic pedicles; SV – Seminal vesicals; C – Clip.

a b c

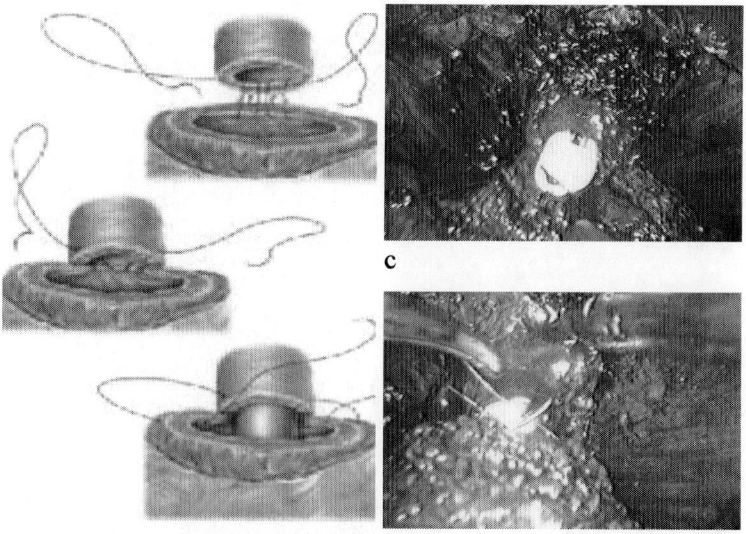

Figure 13. Urethral stump and urethral suture. a. Schematic demontration of continuous suture with two needles. b. Posterior anastomosis completed. c. Anterior anastomosis.

25. The assistant performs the lateral and superior traction of previously mobilized prostate, enabling the clear identification of the prostatic pedicles and the prostate capsular limits. The control of the prostatic pedicles is performed with harmonic or bipolar scalpel in cases without nerve sparing. For complete presevation of neurovascular

bundles polymer or titanium clips (Hem-o-lockÆ) can be used (Figure 12);

26. Exeresis and entrapment of the specimen, placed in the right iliac fossa;
27. Vesicoureteral anastomosis is initiated with the patient in Trendelemburg position in order to improve the visualization of the urethra. The surgeon works with the pararectal 10-mm trocars at the upper end of the table. We perform a running 3-0 polyglecaprone (monocryl) suture with SH needle. We use two 13-cm sutures, one colorless and the other one violet, externally tied by the distal end. A modified van Velthoven suture begins at 4 o'clock position in the bladder directed inwards and each of the sutures rises toward 8 o'clock position, where a single internal knot is made anteriorlly (figure 13) [5];
28. Drainage with Penrose though one of the 5-mm ports;
29. Removal of the specimen by enlargement of the umbilical port and closure of the incisions.

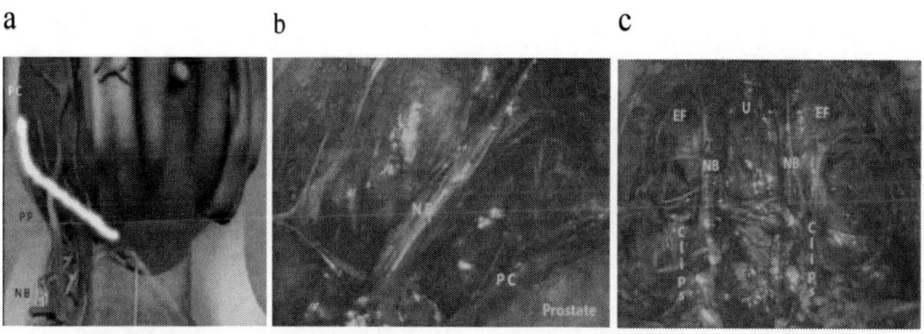

Figure 14. The intrafascial nerve-sparing is the most recent refinement . The dissection plane is near on the prostatic capsule, freeing the prostate laterally from its thin surrounding fascia that contains small vessels and nerves. PC-Prostatic capsule; PP- Prostatic pedicle; NB – Neurovascular bundle; U- Urethra; EF – Endopelvic fascia.

Surgical Steps of Antegrade Technique

The theorical advantage of this technique is to perform the division of dorsal venous plexus as the last surgical step. In this way, less bleeding occurs during initial steps of dissection. The same surgical steps are performed to access the EP cavity. Actually we open the endopelvic fascia only if intrafascial dissection was not elected and the dorsal vein plexus is controlled similar to previously described for retrograde technique. The knot is tied but the plexus is not sectioned, and dissection is performed from the bladder neck to the prostatic apex.

The surgical steps are described below:

1. After tying Santorini's plexus, the back bleeding suture is placed on the anterior surface of the prostate. Traction is placed in this knot to pull the prostate and the bladder through the six (suprapubic) trocar. Beniquet forceps can aid to find the transition between the bladder and prostate. At this moment the bladder neck is opened with harmonic scalpel and cold scissor.
2. The Foley catheter is grasped to perform the posterior bladder neck dissection.
3. After opening the posterior layer of detrusor muscle, vasa deferentia are identified, dissected free and divided. Diagonal contralateral traction is performed to better expose the homolateral seminal vesicle. Here there is always a small artery and a careful dissection is necessary. Vessels near to the vascular bundle are controlled athermically with clips. Seminal vesicles are dissected free.
4. After dissection, both seminal vesicles are retracted anteriorly, the Denonvilliers fascia is opened behind the prostate to identify the perirectal fat and the bundles are dissected gently without any thermic source.
5. Hem-O-lock clips are used to control the pedicles. At this moment we decide about the level of preservation of neurovascular bundle (intrafacial, interfascial or extrafascial) .We should see perfectly well the limits between the prostate and the pedicle. In selected and favorable patients in witch complete preservation is possible we perform the most recent refinement of the endoscopic extraperitoneal radical prostatectomy - the intrafascial nerve-sparing (figure 14). As part of the intrafascial technique, the dissection plane is directly on the prostatic capsule, freeing the prostate laterally from its thin surrounding fascia that contains small vessels and nerves. The technique enables puboprostatic ligament preservation, leaving intact endopelvic fascia, periprostatic fascia, and neurovascular bundles. Based on anatomic relations between investing prostatic fascial layers and the neurovascular bundle, emphasis is placed on division of the apical prostatic urethra between the anterolateral endopelvic fascia and Dennonvilliers fascia in avoidance of the apical nerves. The "Veil

of Aphrodite" is maintained and the visceral fascias opened anteriorly simultaneous with pedicle ligation [31]. Vertical incision in the distal portion of the fused Dennonvilliers layers is necessary to make this dissection atraumatic to the paraprostatic neurovascular bundle.

6. A Beniquet is important to complete lateral dissection of the prostate. It can push the prostate down to favor the dissection between the prostatic apex and bundle.
7. At this moment apical dissection is performed. It is an extremely important step because most positive margin occurs in the apex. Excellent visualization allow better preservation of urinary sphincter maintaining the urethral stump attached to puboprostatic ligament without jeopardize apical margin. The dorsal venous complex is than divided. The urethra and recto-urethralis is finally divided and the specimen freed from last adhesions
8. Pathological specimen is removed in a bag
9. Running vesico-urethral anastomosis is done similar to previous description.

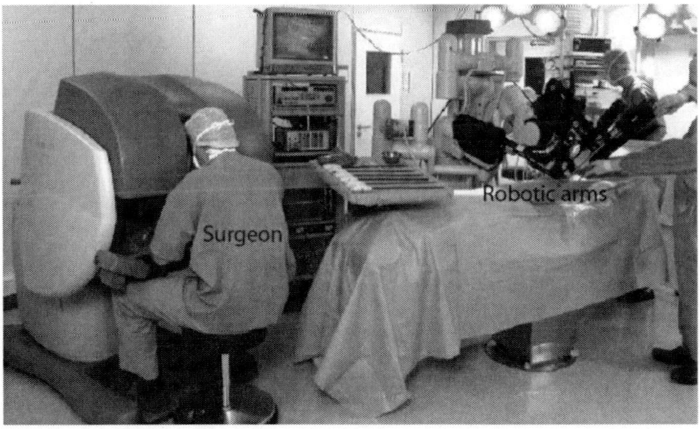

Figure 15. Robotic system consists in a console to the main surgeon manipulation and robotic arms in the surgical field.

Extraperitoneal Robotic Assisted Laparoscopic Surgery (EP-RALP)

Minimally invasive prostatectomies are increasingly common in current urological practice. In such context, robotic assisted laparoscopic surgery

(RALP) is becoming the most performed surgical procedure for prostate cancer in several countries (figure 15). The route for performing RALP, extraperitoneal (EP) vs. transperitoneal (TP), is more a matter of surgeon's preference, even though in a subset of patients one route might allow easier access than the other [32].

Advantages of the TP route include a larger working space, greater facility in viewing anatomical structures and possibly a lower tension in the vesicourethral anastomosis [33]. However, the EP route allows a more similar surgery to open retropubic prostatectomy, maintains the integrity of the peritoneal barrier and therefore bears lesser concerns about postoperative bleeding, urinary leaks, ileum and bowel injury [33]. Another advantage is that the extreme Trendelemburg position can be avoided as the peritoneum helps to retract the bowel [34]. Situations in which the EP route might bring some benefit include obese patients and patients with prior abdominal surgeries.

EP space can be created with balloon dilatators [34], homemade balloon dilatators [33] or dilatating the EP space with the surgeon's fingers and posteriorly with the camera. Veress needles are unnecessary with the EP approach, reducing the risk of bowel injury. To the best of our knowledge, less than 800 of such procedures have been published [35]. However, results seem to be very similar to those obtained through TP route [36] (Table 2)

Robotic surgery have permitted that this difficult operation can be done by a growing number of urologic oncologic surgeons. On the other hand, series comparing pure laparoscopic and robotic radical prostatectomy for groups that have expertise in both techniques have shown that there are no functional or oncological advantage for robotic in experienced hands.

Results of Personal Series and Comparison with Literature Data

Our results with EP-LRP are consistent to those reported in the literature [14,41,42] (table 3). After the 50 initial procedures, we had a mean operative time of 180 minutes, mean blood loss of 210 ml, transfusion rate of 2.25% and no conversion to open surgery. Complication rate occurred in 12.5% of these men and median hospital stay was 2 days. Erection sufficient to penetration in previous potent patients occurred in 75% of men and severe urinary incontinence occurred in 2 % of men. Overall positive surgical margins occurred in 10% of men. In a 3.5-years mean follow-up 90% of patients were free of PSA recurrence.

Table 2. Surgical outcomes of current series of EP-RALP documented [34,35,37-40]

Author	Year	N	PSA recur	6 Mo Continence	6 MoPotency	Op.Time (min)	Complic	EBL (mL)	Transfusion
Madeb	2007	150	-	-	60%	223	-	196	-
Joseph	2006	325	0.6%	96% (no pads)	70%	180	9.8%	196	1.3%
Gettman	2003	4	-	-	-	274	0		0
Esposito	2005	154							
Atug	2006	40	-	-	-	229	12.5%	221	-
John	2007	100	5%	95%	78%	180		300	0

Table 3. Data from early series on EP-LRP [14,24,43-45]

	Stolzenburg 2007	Xue 2007	Cathelineau 2004	Bollens 2002	Tobias-Machado 2008
N cases	1,300	65	100	50	200
Surgical time (min)	153 (50-320)	172 (100-440)	163	317	210
Pre.Op.PSA (ng/ml) *	10.1 ng/ml	10	9.1	-	
Blood Loss (ml)	-	340	375	680	330
Positive margins (%)	34.3	9.2	21	22	10
Major complications	-	1 Rectal injury	0	1 conversion	
Transfusion rate (%)	0.9	10.8	-	-	2.5
Sexual potencyafter 1 year (%)	34	-	-	67	75
Urinary continenceafter 1 year (%)	91.9	89.2**	-	85	90

* Pre operative PSA. ** Continence after 3 months.

Results of Personal Series and Comparison with Literature Data

Our results with EP-LRP are consistent to those reported in the literature [14, 41, 42] (table 3). After the 50 initial procedures, we had a mean operative time of 180 minutes, mean blood loss of 210 ml, transfusion rate of 2.25% and no conversion to open surgery. Complication rate occurred in 12.5% of these men and median hospital stay was 2 days. Erection sufficient to penetration in previous potent patients occurred in 75% of men and severe urinary incontinence occurred in 2 % of men. Overall positive surgical margins occurred in 10% of men. In a 3.5-years mean follow-up 90% of patients were free of PSA recurrence.

Conclusion

Radical prostatectomy is a continually developing technique. In any of the three modalities (open, laparoscopic or robotic) it is consolidated as a first-line treatment for localized prostate cancer [36]. It is still difficult to draw definitive conclusions about the best approach since no conclusive prospective randomized studies comparing the three techniques are available.

Patients' trends may also be considered and it seems clear that the minimum invasive approaches tend to prevail. It has to be stated also that each surgeon has to base on his own results, since the surgeon is definitely the most decisive factor in the operative outcomes.

EP-LRP is efficient, providing the benefits of both laparoscopy and a totally EP approach. Severe complications related to learning curve (urinary and rectal fistula) seem to be less morbid in EP-LRP. However studies demonstrate equivalence between trans and extra peritoneal access in the hands of experienced surgeons. Reduction of complication rate and better oncological and functional outcomes can be achieved with increased surgeon experience. Reduced learning curve period favored RALP to gain acceptance in USA. However costs, availability and training facilities are important issues associated with the acceptance of minimally invasive surgery in developing countries.

When treating a patient with prostate cancer, the main goals are to obtain the cancer cure, rapid recovery of complete urinary continence and preservation of sexual function. Additionally to this triad, we shall also mention that it is also desirable to obtain these results with low morbidity and complication rates. As recent studies have demonstrated, for both LRP and RALP, TP vs. EP routes don't interfere in the results, with similar cure, continence, potency and complication rates. Therefore surgeon preference shall play a role in deciding which approach to be used.

References

[1] Walsh PC, Partin AW, Epstein JI. Cancer control and quality of life following anatomical radical retropubic prostatectomy: results at 10 years. *J. Urol.,* 1994;152(5 Pt 2):1831-6.

[2] Young HH. XV. Cancer of the Prostate: A Clinical, Pathological and Post-Operative Analysis of 111 Cases. *Ann. Surg.,* 1909;50(6):1144-233.

[3] Walsh PC, Donker PJ. Impotence following radical prostatectomy: insight into etiology and prevention. *J. Urol.,* 1982;128(3):492-7.

[4] Catalona WJ, Carvalhal GF, Mager DE, Smith DS. Potency, continence and complication rates in 1,870 consecutive radical retropubic prostatectomies. *J. Urol.,* 1999;162(2):433-8.

[5] Carlin BI, Resnick MI. Anatomic approach to radical perineal prostatectomy. *Urol. Clin. North Am.* 1995;22(2):461-73.

[6] Schuessler WW, Schulam PG, Clayman RV, Kavoussi LR. Laparoscopic radical prostatectomy: initial short-term experience. *Urology* 1997;50(6):854-7.

[7] Guillonneau B, Cathelineau X, Barret E, Rozet F, Vallancien G. Laparoscopic radical prostatectomy: technical and early oncological assessment of 40 operations. *Eur. Urol.,* 1999;36(1):14-20.

[8] Abbou CC, Salomon L, Hoznek A, Antiphon P, Cicco A, Saint F, et al. Laparoscopic radical prostatectomy: preliminary results. *Urology* 2000;55(5):630-4.

[9] Guillonneau B, Vallancien G. Laparoscopic radical prostatectomy: the Montsouris technique. *J. Urol.,* 2000;163(6):1643-9.

[10] Rassweiler J, Sentker L, Seemann O, Hatzinger M, Stock C, Frede T. Heilbronn laparoscopic radical prostatectomy. Technique and results after 100 cases. *Eur. Urol.,* 2001;40(1):54-64.

[11] Raboy A, Ferzli G, Albert P. Initial experience with extraperitoneal endoscopic radical retropubic prostatectomy. *Urology* 1997;50(6): 849-53.

[12] Dubernard P, Benchetrit S, Chaffange P, Hamza T, Van Box Som P. [Retrograde extraperitoneal laparoscopic prostatectomy (R.E.I.P). Simplified technique (based on a series of 143 cases]. *Prog. Urol.* 2003;13(1):163-74.

[13] Berry A, Korkes F, Hu JC. Landmarks for Consistent Nerve-Sparing during Robotic Prostatectomy. *J. Endourol.,* 2008;IN PRESS.

[14] Tobias-Machado M, Forseto P, Jr., Medina JA, Watanabe M, Juliano RV, Wroclawski ER. Laparoscopic radical prostatectomy by extraperitoneal access with duplication of the open technique. *Int. Braz. J. Urol.,* 2004;30(3):221-6.

[15] Box GN, Ahlering TE. Robotic radical prostatectomy: long-term outcomes. *Curr. Opin. Urol.,* 2008;18(2):173-9.

[16] Stein A, deKernion JB, Smith RB, Dorey F, Patel H. Prostate specific antigen levels after radical prostatectomy in patients with organ confined and locally extensive prostate cancer. *J. Urol.,* 1992;147(3 Pt 2):942-6.

[17] Catalona WJ, Smith DS. Cancer recurrence and survival rates after anatomic radical retropubic prostatectomy for prostate cancer: intermediate-term results. *J. Urol.,* 1998;160(6 Pt 2):2428-34.

[18] Kawabata G, Hara I, Hara S, Isotani S, Sakai Y, Wada Y, et al. [Laparoscopic radical prostatectomy: initial 17 case report]. *Nippon Hinyokika Gakkai Zasshi* 2001;92(7):647-55.

[19] Turk I, Deger S, Winkelmann B, Schonberger B, Loening SA. Laparoscopic radical prostatectomy. Technical aspects and experience with 125 cases. *Eur. Urol.,* 2001;40(1):46-52; discussion 53.

[20] Farnham SB, Webster TM, Herrell SD, Smith JA, Jr. Intraoperative blood loss and transfusion requirements for robotic-assisted radical prostatectomy versus radical retropubic prostatectomy. *Urology* 2006;67(2):360-3.

[21] Bhayani SB, Pavlovich CP, Strup SE, Dahl DM, Landman J, Fabrizio MD, et al. Laparoscopic radical prostatectomy: a multi-institutional study of conversion to open surgery. *Urology* 2004;63(1):99-102.

[22] Smith JA, Jr. Outcome after radical prostatectomy depends on surgical technique but not approach. *Curr. Urol. Rep.,* 2002;3(3):179-81.

[23] Stolzenburg JU, Rabenalt R, Do M, Ho K, Dorschner W, Waldkirch E, et al. Endoscopic extraperitoneal radical prostatectomy: oncological and functional results after 700 procedures. *J. Urol.,* 2005;174(4 Pt 1):1271-5; discussion 1275.

[24] Stolzenburg JU, Rabenalt R, Do M, Truss MC, Burchardt M, Herrmann TR, et al. Endoscopic extraperitoneal radical prostatectomy: the

University of Leipzig experience of 1,300 cases. *World J. Urol.* 2007;25(1):45-51.

[25] Su LM, Link RE, Bhayani SB, Sullivan W, Pavlovich CP. Nerve-sparing laparoscopic radical prostatectomy: replicating the open surgical technique. *Urology* 2004;64(1):123-7.

[26] Rozet F, Galiano M, Cathelineau X, Barret E, Cathala N, Vallancien G. Extraperitoneal laparoscopic radical prostatectomy: a prospective evaluation of 600 cases. *J. Urol.,* 2005;174(3):908-11.

[27] Humphreys MR, Gettman MT, Chow GK, Zincke H, Blute ML. Minimally invasive radical prostatectomy.*Mayo Clin Proc* 2004;79(9):1169-80.

[28] Gettman MT, Blute ML. Critical comparison of laparoscopic, robotic, and open radical prostatectomy: techniques, outcomes, and cost. *Curr. Urol. Rep.,* 2006;7(3):193-9.

[29] Guillonneau B, el-Fettouh H, Baumert H, Cathelineau X, Doublet JD, Fromont G, et al. Laparoscopic radical prostatectomy: oncological evaluation after 1,000 cases a Montsouris Institute. *J. Urol.,* 2003;169(4):1261-6.

[30] Tobias-Machado M, Lasmar MT, Medina JJ, Forseto PH, Jr., Juliano RV, Wroclawski ER. Preliminary experience with extraperitoneal endoscopic radical prostatectomy through duplication of the open technique. *Int. Braz. J. Urol.,* 2005;31(3):228-35.

[31] Curto F, Benijts J, Pansadoro A, Barmoshe S, Hoepffner JL, Mugnier C, et al. Nerve sparing laparoscopic radical prostatectomy: our technique. *Eur. Urol.,* 2006;49(2):344-52.

[32] Ficarra V, Cavalleri S, Novara G, Aragona M, Artibani W. Evidence from robot-assisted laparoscopic radical prostatectomy: a systematic review. *Eur. Urol.,* 2007;51(1):45-55; discussion 56.

[33] Tobias-Machado M, Juliano RV, Gaspar HA, Rocha RP, Borrelli M, Wroclawski ER. Videoendoscopic surgery by extraperitoneal access: technical aspects and indication. *Int Braz J Urol* 2003;29(5):441-9.

[34] Joseph JV, Rosenbaum R, Madeb R, Erturk E, Patel HR. Robotic extraperitoneal radical prostatectomy: an alternative approach. *J. Urol.* 2006;175(3 Pt 1):945-50; discussion 951.

[35] John H, Schmid DM, Fehr JL. [Extraperitoneal radical prostatectomy Da Vinci]. *Actas. Urol. Esp.* 2007;31(6):580-6.

[36] Badani KK, Kaul S, Menon M. Evolution of robotic radical prostatectomy: assessment after 2766 procedures. *Cancer* 2007;110(9):1951-8.

[37] Atug F, Castle EP, Woods M, Srivastav SK, Thomas R, Davis R. Transperitoneal versus extraperitoneal robotic-assisted radical prostatectomy: is one better than the other? *Urology* 2006;68(5):1077-81.

[38] Madeb R, Golijanin D, Knopf J, Vicente I, Erturk E, Patel HR, et al. Patient-reported validated functional outcome after extraperitoneal robotic-assisted nerve-sparing radical prostatectomy. *Jsls* 2007;11(4):443-8.

[39] Gettman MT, Hoznek A, Salomon L, Katz R, Borkowski T, Antiphon P, et al. Laparoscopic radical prostatectomy: description of the extraperitoneal approach using the da Vinci robotic system. *J. Urol.* 2003;170(2 Pt 1):416-9.

[40] Esposito MP, Ilbeigi P, Ahmed M, Lanteri V. Use of fourth arm in da Vinci robot-assisted extraperitoneal laparoscopic prostatectomy: novel technique. *Urology* 2005;66(3):649-52.

[41] Tobias-Machado M, Juliano RV, Tristão RA, Watanabe M, Forseto Jr PH and Wroclawski ER. Laparoscopic prostatectomy: Comparative study beetwen transperitoneal and extraperitoneal approachs during learning curve. *Einstein* 2007; 5(3): 203-208.

[42] Tobias-Machado M, Starling ES, Juliano RV, Tavares A, Wroclawski ER. Learning curve improves functional and oncological outcomes on pure laparoscopic prostatectomy: experience of a reference center in Brazil. *Urology* 2008 (in press).

[43] Xue BX, Shan YX, Abbou CC. [Extraperitoneal laparoscopic radical prostatectomy for prostate cancer: a report of 65 cases]. *Zhonghua Nan Ke Xue* 2007;13(11):1012-5.

[44] Cathelineau X, Cahill D, Widmer H, Rozet F, Baumert H, Vallancien G. Transperitoneal or extraperitoneal approach for laparoscopic radical prostatectomy: a false debate over a real challenge. *J. Urol.,* 2004;171(2 Pt 1):714-6.

[45] Bollens R, Vanden Bossche M, Roumeguere T, Damoun A, Ekane S, Hoffmann P, et al. Extraperitoneal laparoscopic radical prostatectomy. Results after 50 cases. *Eur. Urol.,* 2001;40(1):65-9.

In: Prostatectomies
Editors: H. Alvelos and Y. Izidoro

ISBN: 978-1- 62081-077-4
© 2012 Nova Science Publishers, Inc.

Chapter VIII

PSA Nadir Post-Radical Prostatectomy Might Predict Long-Term Biochemical Recurrence*

Fernando Korkes[1] and André Costa-Matos[2]
[1]ABC Medical School – São Paulo, Brazil
[2]5th year Urology resident – São Paulo, Brazil

Abstract

Radical prostatectomy is the most widely applied treatment for localized prostate cancer. Postoperative PSA levels are expected to be close to zero and PSA levels above 0.2 ng/dL generally characterize recurrence. However, there is no consensual definition for PSA levels to define cure after radical prostatectomy yet. The aim of the present study was to evaluate post prostatectomy PSA level and its association with prostate cancer relapse.

Methods: A hundred and six men (median=64.0±6.9 years, range 49-80 years) with localized prostate cancer underwent radical retropubic

* A version of this chapter also appears in *PSA and Prostate Cancer*, edited by Jake A. Saylor and Lionel B. Michaels, published by Nova Science Publishers, Inc. It was submitted for appropriate modifications in an effort to encourage wider dissemination of research.

prostatectomy were followed between 1996 and 2006, for a minimum 24-month follow up (mean 46.5 months). Postoperative ultrasensitive PSA levels were assessed after 30 days, every 3 months for the first two years and twice a year thereafter. Patients were divided in four groups according to postoperative PSA nadir: Group 1 (<0.04 ng/dL); group 2 (0.04-0.09 ng/dL); group 3 (0.09 –0.2 ng/dL); and group 4 (>0.2 ng/dL). *Results:* Sixty-two men (66.0%) had postoperative PSA <0.04 ng/dl, of whom 30.6% presented biochemical relapse after a median of 44.4±17.4 months. Almost all men that had postoperative PSA nadir above 0.04 ng/dl presented biochemical recurrence, 100% and 90.3% for PSA 0.04-0.09 ng/dL and >0.09 ng/dL respectively (x^2=24.96; p<0.0001).

Conclusions: Biochemical recurrence after RP is normally defined as PSA level above 0.2 ng/dl, based on studies prior to application of ultrasensitive PSA assays. However, patients with PSA nadir between 0.04-0.2 ng/dL have demonstrated a 91% chance of biochemical recurrence. These patients might benefit of additional treatments, such as adjuvant radiation therapy, with probably more benefits that patients with positive surgical margins, as they have higher probability of disease progression (91% vs. 69%). In conclusion, men with detectable PSA after RP must be follow closely, and adjuvant treatments might be considered.

Introduction

Radical prostatectomy is the gold standard treatment for localized prostate cancer, and has been proven to provide excellent long-term cancer control in patients with pathologically organ confined disease. Although other treatments as radiotherapy, brachiterapy and crioterapy have also been applied with success, surgery remains the most applied treatment, with many advantages for low-risk patients.

Follow up is easier, with consensual definitions of PSA relapse and the option of radiotherapy in cases of postoperative biochemical recurrence is easier than surgery after radiotherapy. Postoperative PSA level are expected to be close to zero and recurrence is characterized by PSA levels above 0,2 ng/dl [1]. However, there is no consensual definition for PSA levels to define cure after radical prostatectomy.

Previous studies have suggested an associaton between detectable postprostatectomy PSA with biochemical failure[2]. The aim of the present study was to evaluate postprostatectomy ultrasensible PSA level and its association with prostate cancer relapse.

Patients and Methods

A hundred and six men (median=64±6.9 years, range 49-80 years) with localized prostate cancer underwent radical retropubic prostatectomy were followed between 1996 and 2006. PSA was accessed 30 days after surgery, after 3 months during the first two years and twice a year thereafter. All patients had a minimum of two years of follow up. Patients were divided in four groups according to postoperative PSA nadir: Group 1 (<0.04); group 2 (0.04- 0.09); group 3 (0.09 – 0.2); group 4 (>0.2). Biochemical relapse was determined after at least two consecutive raises in PSA level above 0.2 ng/dl or when a second-line treatment was initiated. Demographics data, PSA values, and prognostic factors were evaluated and are listed in tables 1 and 2.

Table 1. Preoperative clinical and patological features, demographic data, blood loss and transfusion rates

Age	64 ± 6.8 - (49-80)	
Clinical stage	T1b – 2 (3.7%) T1c - 27 (50.0%) T2a - 54 (46.3%)	
PSA	11.8 ± 11.57	
Prostate weigth	41.7 ± 20.5	
Gleason	2 – 1 (1.1%) 3 – 2 (2.2%) 4 – 1 (1.1%) 5 – 4 (4.3%)	6 – 49 (52.7%) 7 – 28 (30.1%) 8 – 7 (7.5%) 9 – 1 (1.1%)
Bleeding	865 ± 437 (175 – 2000) ml	
Transfusion rate	1.5 ± 1.1 (0 - 4) UI	

Table 2. Biochemical recurrence according to patological findings

	Present	Absent	P
Vascular invasion	10/16 (62.5%)	27/67 (40.3%)	0.108
Perineural invasion	24/44(54.5%)	14/38 (36.8%)	0.109
Seminal vesicle invasion	13/15 (86.7%)	33/77 (42.89%)	0.002
Lymph node invasion	2/3 (66.7%)	40/84 (47.6%)	0.517
Urethral Margin +	10/12 (83.3%)	30/74 (40.5%)	0.006
Vesical Margin +	3/6 (50.0%)	35/77 (45.5%)	0.830
Capsule invasion	18/25 (72.0%)	26/64 (40.6%)	0.008

Table 3. Patients' evolution after RP according to postoperative PSA level

PSA	Free of disease	Recurrence	Total
<0.04	43 (69.4%)	19 (30.6%)	62
0.04-0.09	0 (0%)	2 (100%)	2
>0.09	3 (9.7%)	28 (90.3%)	31
Total	46 (48.4%)	49 (51.6%)	95

(x^2=24.96; p<0.0001).

Statistical analysis was performed in SPSS program and significance was considered at p <0.05.

Results

Sixty-two men (66%) had postoperative PSA <0.04 ng/dl and 30.6% presented biochemical relapse after a median time of 44.4±17.4 months. Biochemical recurrence rates for men with PSA 0.04-0.09, 0.91-0.20 and >0.20 ng/dl were respectively 100%, 92.9% and 88.2% (x^2=24.96; p<0.0001, see table 3).

Of men with PSA<0.04 with biochemical recurrence vs. without recurrence, 8 (61.5%) vs. 6 (16.2%) had locally advanced disease (p<0.002). Pathological features associated with relapse included seminal vesicle invasion, positive urethral margin and extraprostatic disease (Table 2). Patients with at least one of these factors had higher recurrence rates (70.2%, n=33 vs. 31%, n=9; p< 0,01). Table 1 demonstrates demographic data, pathological features, blood loss and transfusion rates.

Discussion

Despite the knowledge that biochemical recurrence after RP is defined only with PSA level above 0.2ng/dl, our data shows that detectable PSA post surgery is associated with more recurrence rates. Shen et al studied the serum PSA nadir after RP in 906 men followed for one year[2]. Men with a nadir of less than 0.01 ng/ml had a significantly lower relapse rate (4%) than men with a nadir of 0.01 (12%) (p <0.01), 0.02 (16%) (p <0.025) or 0.04 or greater ng/ml (89%) (p <0.01). They used an ultrasensitive assay for detecting PSA.

We have found similar results after a longer follow up period, with recurrence for PSA >0.04 of 91% and 30.6% for PSA <0.04 ng/dl.

On the other hand, is known the benign evolution of some patients with PSA between 0.2 and 0.5ng/dl, of whom 10% do not present with recurrence[3]. In our study, 12% of patients with PSA >0.2 were free of disease after a median time of 46.5 months. This might occur due to peripheral glands near vesical neck that are left in the surgery.

As much as 50% of patients with positive surgical margins progresses[4]. In our data, patients who had this patological feature had a recurrence rate of 69%, situation in which salvage radiation therapy might be bennefical [3,5]. However 31% of these men with positive surgical margins would have received unnecessary radiation. Stephenson and coworkers demonstrated that salvage radiation therapy has better results when it is done with PSA<0.5 with 48% (95% CI, 40% to 56%) of patients treated with salvage radiation therapy alone were free of disease at 6 years [3,6]. This suggests that close follow up and PSA dynamics might be observed. In our study, most men with PSA >0.04 (91%) demonstrated biochemical recurrence, and could probably benefit from adjuvant therapies.

Conclusion

Our study suggests that patients with detectable PSA after RP must be followed closely, and even men with PSA levels bellow 0.2 ng/dl might in the future present with biochemical recurrence. Additionally, ultrasensitive PSA level > 0.04 ng/dl after surgery, as positive surgical margins, might predict recurrence and consequentily guide adjuvant radiotherapy.

References

[1] Amling, CL; Bergstralh, EJ; Blute, ML; Slezak, JM; Zincke, H. Defining prostate specific antigen progression after radical prostatectomy: what is the most appropriate cut point? *J. Urol.*, 2001, 165, 1146-51,

[2] Shen, S; Lepor, H; Yaffee, R; Taneja, SS. Ultrasensitive serum prostate specific antigen nadir accurately predicts the risk of early relapse after radical prostatectomy. *J. Urol.*, 2005, 173, 777-80,

[3] Stephenson, AJ; Scardino, PT; Kattan, MW; Pisansky, TM; Slawin, KM; Klein, EA; Anscher, MS; Michalski, JM; Sandler, HM; Lin, DW. et al. Predicting the outcome of salvage radiation therapy for recurrent prostate cancer after radical prostatectomy. *J. Clin. Oncol.,* 2007, 25, 2035-41.

[4] Karakiewicz, PI; Eastham, JA; Graefen, M; Cagiannos, I; Stricker, PD; Klein, E; Cangiano, T; Schroder, FH; Scardino, PT; Kattan, MW. Prognostic impact of positive surgical margins in surgically treated prostate cancer: multi-institutional assessment of 5831 patients. *Urology.,* 66, 1245-50, 2005.

[5] Thompson, IM; Jr., Tangen, CM; Paradelo, J; Lucia, MS; Miller, G; Troyer, D; Messing, E; Forman, J; Chin, J; Swanson, G; et al. Adjuvant radiotherapy for pathologically advanced prostate cancer: a randomized clinical trial. *Jama.,* 296, 2329-35, 2006.

[6] Stephenson, AJ; Kattan, MW; Eastham, JA; Dotan, ZA; Bianco, FJ; Jr., Lilja, H; Scardino, PT. Defining biochemical recurrence of prostate cancer after radical prostatectomy: a proposal for a standardized definition. *J. Clin. Oncol.,* 2006, 24, 3973-8.

Index

D

E

F

K

L

M

N

O

P

Q

R

S

T

U

V

W

Z